Dedicated to

Our Parents

FOREWORD

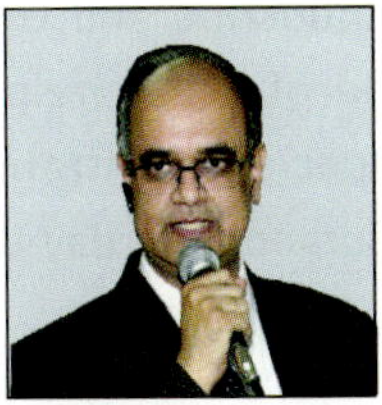

It gives me great privilege to write the foreword for the book **CONCISE CANCER MANUAL** written by Dr. Prashant Rao and Dr. Sarika Mayekar Rao. Both of them were the distinguished post graduate students in the Department of General Surgery at Lokmanya Tilak Municipal Medical College & General Hospital, Sion, Mumbai. They happened to work in my unit during their General Surgery residency. They are extremely talented, sincere and hardworking resident surgeons. They passed their Master's degree with flying colours. Dr Sarika also received Gold medal for coming first in the institution.

In department of General Surgery in LTMMC & GH, we operate about 3500 to 3800 patients in the elective surgical OT per year, out of which about 1000 to 1200 patients are of various cancers. Although cancer surgery and oncology have become exclusive branches of surgery with their super specialty degrees after M.S., large number of these patients are treated in General Surgery department of this as well as in many medical colleges of the country. The department of General Surgery in LTMMC & GH is known to offer a comprehensive treatment to the patients of various cancers with pre and post-operative chemotherapy at the same place.

A student appearing for M.S. General Surgery exam is expected to know in depth, about all types of cancers. Reading exhaustively about every cancer could be difficult for an exam going student. The **CONCISE CANCER MANUAL** will help the students to understand basic points about every cancer. The book contents are spread into 4 important sections namely GIT, HPB, Endocrine and Genitourinary cancers. This book will undoubtedly be of great help for not only theory as well as viva-voce and speciality entrance examinations but also to practising General Surgeons in day-to-day management of cancer patients.

I compliment Dr. Prashant and Dr. Sarika for their painstaking efforts to write this book and I hope that their sincere and earnest efforts would be truly rewarded.

Happy Reading!

Dr. Mohan A. Joshi
M.S., F.C.P.S., F.A.I.S., M.N.A.M.S.

Professor & Head, Department of General Surgery
Consultant GI Surgeon
Advanced Therapeutic Endoscopist,
Lokmanya Tilak Municipal Medical College & General Hospital,
Sion (W), Mumbai - 400022.

24th October, 2017

ACKNOWLEDGEMENT

We would like to thank for all the teachings and help,

- Dr. Mohan A Joshi, Dr. Minakshi G and all our Seniors and friends from our Alma mater, LTMMC, Sion, Mumbai,
- Dr. Satish Dharap, Dr. R M Joshi and all our Seniors and friends from TNMC & Nair Hospital, Mumbai,
- Dr. Avinash Supe, Dr. Vinita Puri, Dr. Kapil Agarwal, Dr. Nilesh, Dr. Deepak and all our Seniors & friends from Seth GSMC and KEM Hospital, Mumbai,
- Dr. Satheesh Iype, Dr. Shaji P, Dr. N P Kamalesh, Dr. Pramil K, Dr. Rohan, Dr. Kartik and Dr. Prasanna from PVS Memorial Hospital, Kochi, Kerala.

Special thanks to Dr. Paresh Vohra, Dr. Adarsh Puranik, Ashish Arts and our family for the constant support.

Also, special thanks to Mr. Rajesh Bhalani from Bhalani Publishers, Mumbai and Mr. Satish Kumar Jain from CBS Publishers & Distributors, New Delhi for their constant support, encouragement and speedy publication of an excellent quality.

Lastly, I would like to thank all the readers and all the best for the forthcoming examinations.

CONTENTS

Section - I

Gastro-Intestinal Oncology

Section - II

Hepato-Pancreatico-Biliary Oncology

Section - III

Genito-Urinary Oncology

Section - IV

Endocrinological Oncology

SECTION I

Gastro-Intestinal Oncology

Chapter 1

Carcinoma Esophagus

INTRODUCTION:

- Male > Female
- M/C 5th decade onwards
- Incidence increases with age.
- M/C in middle 3rd of esophagus.
- Incidence in lower 3rd of esophagus is rising.

HISTOLOGY:

- Squamous cell Carcinoma →

  More in upper & middle third of esophagus. M/C type worldwide, chemo radiation sensitive, exophytic.

- Adeno Carcinoma ›

  Mainly affects lower third, mainly whites. M/C type in the US, less sensitive to chemo radiation, infiltrative.

ETIOLOGY:

- Smoking
- Alcoholism
- Dietary factors → Smoked & salted food contains high amount of Nitrosamine which is carcinogenic
- Nutritional deficiency → Vitamins : A & C

  Mineral : Molybdenum and Zinc
- Repeated mucosal trauma :

  a. Ingestion of hot liquids

b. Achalasia cardia.

c. Diverticula.

d. Caustic ingestion.

- External beam radiation.
- Human Papilloma Virus (HPV).
- Premalignant conditions :

a. Plummer - Wilsons syndrome
(Iron deficiency anemia + glossitis + esophageal web).

b. Tylosis.

c. Other cancers of aero digestive tract : (concept of field cancerization).

- Helicobacter Pylori (H. pylori) CAG-A strain is a risk factor for SCC.
- Obesity is protective against SCC.
- For Adenocarcinoma :

a. GERD → Barrett's esophagus → dysplasia → Adenocarcinoma.

b. Obesity.

c. H. pylori CAG-A strain is protective.

Whatever the histological type, in view of the fact that esophagus has only 2 layers, with a rich vascular and lymphatic supply, esophageal cancers are bound to be highly aggressive.

SIGNS/SYMPTOMS :

- Majority presents with DYSPHAGIA with WEIGHT LOSS which are indicators of an advanced disease. Thcsc symptoms usually starts after $2/3^{rd}$ of the esophageal lumen gets compromised.

- Choking, coughing & Aspiration suggests-Tracheo-esophageal fistula.
- Hoarseness of voice suggests-Recurrent Laryngeal Nerve infiltration.
- Early disease is usually asymptomatic OR mimics GERD-main reason for the late detection.
- M/C site of distant metastasis : Liver > lung > bone.

DIAGNOSIS :

1. **Esophagogram/Barium swallow is the preferred First test for any patient with dysphagia.**
   - It can identify subtle mucosal changes as well as describe gross tumour morphology
   - Characteristic appearance in carcinoma : Apple core deformity, Rat tail deformity
2. **Upper GI Endoscopy :**
   - Describes Site, extent, nature & provides tissue for Biopsy
   - Provides information regarding location in relation to cricopharyngeus & GEJ
   - Endoscopy with biopsy is investigation of choice for diagnosis
3. **Computerised Tomography :**
   - Provides information regarding Loco-regional stage as well as presence or absence of Abdominal Metastasis
4. **Positron Emission Tomography :**
   - Role not clearly established
   - Can identify occult metastasis not detected on CT.

- However it has No role in early cancer as it does not detect tumour < 10 mm & tumour invasion.
- Local nodes are not seen separately from primary unless they are at a distant site. Inflammatory lymph nodes may also appear positive on PET.

5. **MRI :**

Not routinely performed nor advised in Ca esophagus.

6. **Endoscopic Ultra-Sound (EUS) :**
   - Most critical component of staging.
   - investigation of choice for staging
   - T stage & local N stage identified accurately
   - FIVE Layers seen on EUS are as follows :
     - Mucosa : Hyperechoic
     - Muscularis Mucosa : Hypoechoic
     - Submucosa : Hyperechoic
     - Muscularis Propria : Hypoechoic
     - Adventitia : Hyperechoic
   - Nodes < 10 mm is less accurately defined.

7. **Endoscopic mucosal resection (EMR) & Endoscopic submucosal dissection (ESD) :** apart from providing tissue for biopsy, it is potentially therapeutic

8. Bronchoscopy
9. Mediastinoscopy
10. VATS
11. Laproscopy

} for staging & assessing operability

STAGING :

AJCC'S TNM STAGING SYSTEM IS USED

T stage : (Fig. 1.1)

T1 : Tumour invades submucosa.

T2 : Tumour invades muscularis propria.

T3 : Tumour invades adventitia.

T4 : Tumour invading adjacent structures.

N stage :

N1 : Metastasis to 1-2 Lymph Nodes (LN).

N2 : Metastasis to 3-6 Lymph Nodes (LN).

N3 : Metastasis to > 7 Lymph Nodes (LN).

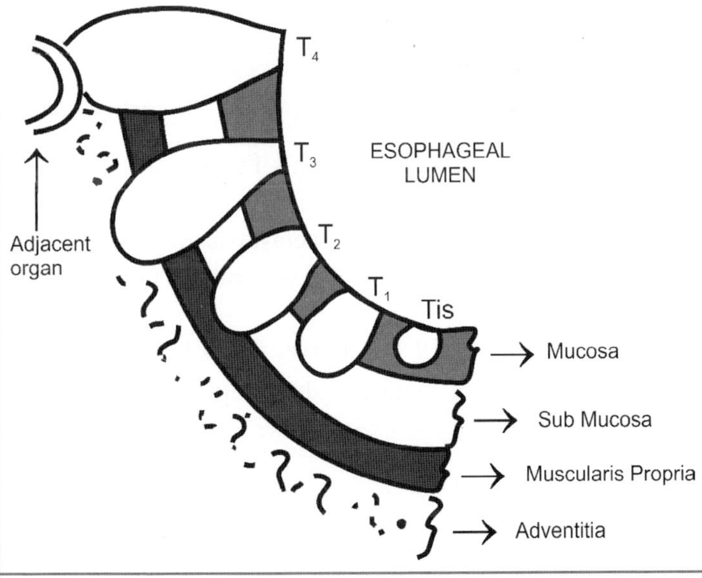

Fig. 1.1: TNM staging for Ca. esophagus

M stage :

M0 : No distant metastasis.

M1 : Distant metastasis present.

ELLIS CLASSIFICATION :

W0 : Tumor going up to Muscularis Mucosa.

W1 : Submucosa & Muscularis propria breached.

W2 : Adventitia infiltrated.

PROGNOSIS :

- Depends on
  - ➢ Depth of infiltration and
  - ➢ Lymph node status
- More the depth of infiltration → Higher the chances of LN invasion
- W0/T1 tumours usually have → No LN invasion

TREATMENT :

- Treatment requires a multimodality approach.
- Evaluate tumour stage & patients fitness for surgery.
- If tumour is well localised, not involving vital structures with no evidence of distant metastasis & if clinical and nutritional status is adequate → treat surgically with a curative intent.
- Resection margin: **10 cm above, 5 cm below.**
- If advanced/distant disease with multiple comorbidities → palliation.

Stage wise treatment :

Stage I : T1 N0 : Surgery alone

If Nodes positive on histopathology → Adjuvant chemo radiation

Stage II : T2/T3 N0 : Neo Adjuvant chemo radiation Followed by Surgery

Stage III : T3 N1/T4 N0 : Neo Adjuvant chemo radiation Followed by Surgery

FACTORS taken into consideration :

1) **Histology :**

- Squamous Cell Ca → are more chemo–radio sensitive than Adenocarcinoma.

2) **Location :**

- ***Cervical tumours*** are usually aggressive.
  - ➢ Bronchoscopy & Endoscopy are essential part of work up.
  - ➢ Neo Adjuvant Chemo-Radiation followed by cervical exploration & Segmental resection.
- ***Upper/Mid thoracic tumours :***
  - ➢ Near total Esophagectomy through thoracotomy or thoracoscopy
- ***Lower esophageal tumours :***
  - ➢ With no Barretts → Distal esophagectomy. via trans Abdominal/trans thoracic approach.
  - ➢ With Barretts → Total/near total esophagectomy. via trans Abdominal/trans thoracic approach.

3) **Depth of invasion :**

T1 :

➢ No role of chemo radiation/Radical lymphadenectomy.

- Surgery alone (Conservative surgery).

  OR

  EMR or ESD for intra mucosal tumours.

T2 :

- Treatment is Controversial.
- > 50% chance of Lymph Node invasion.
- Neo Adjuvant Chemo-Radiation followed by surgery preferred.
- Surgical options :

  En-block Esophagectomy with Radical lymphadenectomy

  Vs.

  Conservative Esophageal resection with Adjuvant Chemotherapy

T3 :

Neo Adjuvant chemo radiation f/b Surgery

T4 :

- Surgery only if no evidence of distant LN or systemic metastasis
- Distant LN/systemic disease

  OR

  Poor nutritional status (Albumin <3.5) with comorbidities } definitive chemo radiation plus palliation

SURGERIES :

1) **Trans Hiatal Esophagectomy (THE) (Orringers): (Fig. 1.2)**
   - Safest of all.

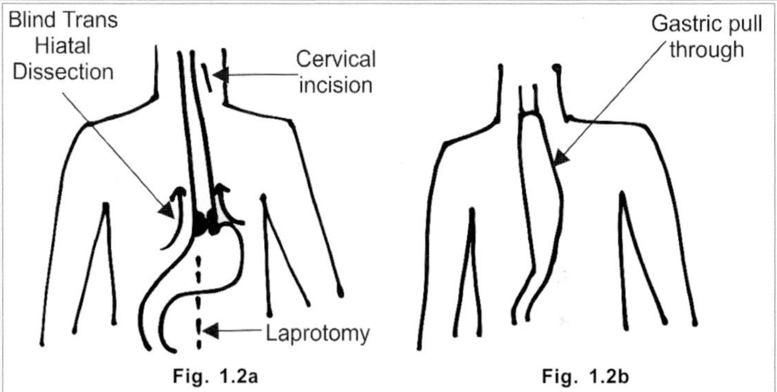

Fig. 1.2: Trans Hiatal Esophagectomy (THE)

- Starting with laparotomy (Abdominal incision) f/b cervical exploration.
- Lymph Nodes in Abdomen, neck & Lower chest removed.

Advantage :

- Reduced cardio pulmonary morbidity.
- Cervical Anastomosis → decreased leak rates & if it does occur, is less morbid.
- Less blood loss with decreased operative time.

Disadvantage :

- Chances of injury to mediastinal structures due to blind dissection.
- Lymph Node clearance may not be adequate.

2) Trans Thoracic Esophagectomy (Ivor Lewis procedure) :

- First operation described for Ca Esophagus.

- Starting with laparotomy (feeding Jejunostomy also done in this phase) f/b Right thoracotomy.
- Transection at level of Azygous vein.
- Anastomosis is Intra thoracic.

Advantage :

- Anastomotic leak rate is lowest.

Disadvantage :

- High cardio pulmonary morbidity.
- Leak can result in sepsis & death.

3) **En-block three field Esophagectomy (Mc Evans procedure) :**

- Most extensive surgery for Ca Esophagus.
- Involves Laparotomy, thoracotomy and cervical exploration
- Involves Radical thoracic & Abdominal lymphadenectomy with wide resection of tissues around the tumor.
- Cervical Esophago-gastric Anastomosis.
- High Cardio-Pulmonary morbidity & leak rates.
- It is of survival advantage if < 9 nodes positive.

4) **Vagal sparing Esophagectomy**

5) **Minimally invasive Esophagectomy**

- Minimally invasive Thoraco-laparoscopic esophagectomy is becoming popular.
- TIME trial has shown MIS to have better short term outcomes such as reduced cardio-pulmonary morbidity compared to open approach

- Long-term oncological outcome is comparabe to open approach

Anastomotic technique : May be Hand sewn or stapled.

Conduit :

- *Stomach is conduit of choice*
- *Other Option :*
  - Colonic Interposition
  - Jejunal Interposition
  - Shorter Interposition : free jejunal patch/forearm flap
- *Conduit position :*
  - Best & shortest : Posterior mediastinum

    OR :
  - Substernal → Preferred if post mediastinum is scarred
  - Right pleural space
  - Subcutaneous

Chemo-Radiation : 5FU + Cisplatin + epirubicin (ECF)
Radiation used : 4500 cgy

- Average survival in advanced disease : 6 months.

Palliative measures :

- Photodynamic therapy
- Laser therapy
- Stenting
  (Self Expansile Metallic Stent : SEMS)

} for dysphagia

- Gastrostomy/Jejunostomy – for nutritional supplementation

Management of Recurrence

- Operable recurrence → Surgery
- Upper GI bleed → laser ablation
- Debilitated → Supportive
- T-O fistula → Stenting
- Systemic spread → Chemo

Special Mention:

Dysphagia Grades :

I. Eating normally

II. Requires liquids with solid meals

III. Able to take semisolid diet

IV. Liquids only

V. Only saliva

VI. None

✡✡✡

Chapter 2 Carcinoma Stomach

- M > F
- M/C in 7th decade
- Worldwide 4th M/C cancer, 2nd M/C leading cause of cancer death
- Japan has highest Ca stomach density
- M/C site in stomach : Antrum

ETIOLOGY :

1) **H. Pylori Infection**

H. Pylori Infection → Chronic gastritis → Gastric Atropy → Intestinal metaplasia → Dysplasia → Carcinoma

- ➢ H pylori causes alteration in P53 & microsatellite instability.
- ➢ High IL-1 → more risk.
- ➢ Cag-A positive → more risk.

2) **Dietary & lifestyle factors :**

- ➢ Salted & smoked food → high in Nitrosamine which is carcinogenic.
- ➢ Lack of fresh fruits & vegetables in diet. They contain Ascorbic Acid which neutralises the harmful Nitroso compounds & O_2 free radicals.
- ➢ Lack of refrigeration.
- ➢ Smoking, not alcohol.

3) Hereditary :

1) Hereditary diffuse gastric Ca resulting from mutation in E-Cadherin gene.

2) Li fraumeni Syndrome.

3) Familial Adenomatous Polyposis (FAP)

4) Hereditary NonPolyposis Colorectal Cancer (HNPCC)

4) Pernicious Anaemia :

Achlorhydria
↓
Gastric Atropy
↓
Intestinal metaplasia ⟶ Dysplasia
↑
Carcinoma

5) Polyp :

➢ Adenomatous polyp carry high risk of carcinomatous transformation.

Suggested treatement :

- Pedunculated polyp → Endoscopic removal.
- Sessile polyp/> 2 cm → Surgical excision.

➢ Fundic gland polyp are usually benign.

But may harbour Adenomatous changes in FAP cases.

6) PPI:

➢ Role controversial

leads to Achlorhydria & allows H. pylori growth

↓

Chronic gastritis → Gastric Atropy → Intestinal metaplasia → Dysplasia → Carcinoma

7) Previous gastric resection with gastro-enteric anastomosis
8) Menetriers disease
9) Blood group A
10) Epstein Barr virus

PROTECTIVE factors :

Aspirin, Vitamin A & C, selenium, zinc, iron, fresh fruits & vegetables.

PATHOLOGY :

Borrmans Classification, based on gross Appearance **(Fig. 2.1)**

Type I → Protruding

Type II → Fungating

Type III → Ulcerative

Type IV → Infiltrative

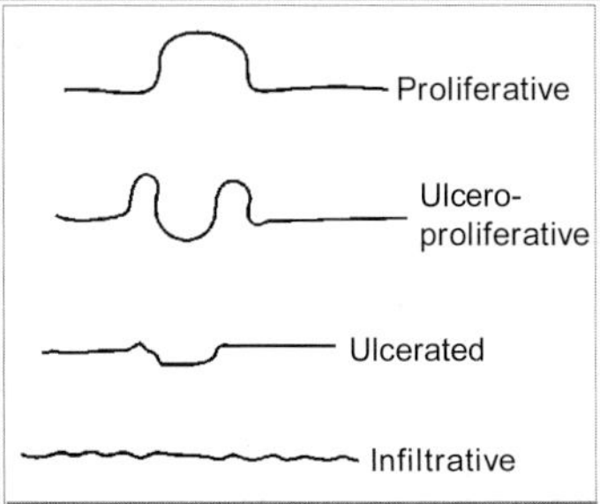

Fig. 2.1: Borrmans Classification

Japanese Endoscopic Society Classification, based on gross Appearance

Type I → Polypoidal

Type II → Superficial

Type III → Ulcerative

Laurens Classification based on histology

Intestinal type	**Diffuse type**
1) Environmental	Familial
2) M > F	F > M / Blood group A
3) Old age predisposed	Young age predisposed
4) Gastric atrophy → Intestinal metaplasia → Dysplasia → Adenocarcinoma →	Signet ring cells present with Poor differentiation
5) P53 P16 inactivation	P53, P16 inactivation
6) **APC** gene mutation	Increase **E-CADHERIN**
7) Distal stomach commonly involved	Proximal stomach
8) Hematogenous spread common	Lymphatic and transmoral spread with intraperitoneal metastasis

WHO Classification based on histology

- Adeno Carcinoma → Papillary, Tubular, Mucinous, Signet ring
- Squamous cell carcinoma
- Adenosquamous carcinoma
- Undifferentiated
- Unclassified

Cancer Genetics :

M/C genetic abnormalities seen with : P-53 & COX-2 genes.

SIGNS/SYMPTOMS :

➢ Pain & weight loss (M/C)

- ➢ Nausea & vomiting
- ➢ Hematemesis / Malena
- ➢ Anorexia, early satiety
- ➢ Weakness

- Proximal tumours tend to cause dysphagia.
- Distal tumours tend to cause GOO (Gastric Outlet Obstruction).
- Usually presents in advanced stages because early symptoms are usually non-specific and wrongly labelled and treated as peptic ulcer disease.

Signs of Advanced disease :

- Virchow's left supraclavicular lymph node
  Irish axillary lymph node
  Sister Mary Joseph umbilical nodule
- Intra Abdominal : ➢ Hepatomegaly
  ➢ Jaundice
  ➢ Ascitis
- Pelvic Examination : ➢ Krukenbergs ovarian tumour (Drop metastasis)
- Blummers shelf on PR examination
- M/C site of distant metastasis : Liver > lung > bone

DIAGNOSTIC TOOLS AND STAGING WORK-UP :

1. Oesophago-Gastro-Duodenoscopy (OGD) and Endoscopic Ultra-Sound (EUS)

- OGD : Describes Site, extent, nature & provides tissue for Biopsy.
- EUS :
  ➢ Helps in T and N staging.

- ➢ One of most important use is that it differentiates HIGH RISK from LOW RISK disease thus helping in prognostification (described later).

2. CT :

- Primary role is in identifying Metastatic disease.
- Less accurate than EUS in Loco-regional (T & N) staging.

3. PET :

- Not a standard staging modality for Gastric cancer. however
- PET avid patients tends to have an aggressive disease
- PET Response to Neo-adjuvant chemotherapy suggests good response

4. **Staging Laproscopy :** Integral part of staging work-up

- Avoids non-therapeutic Laprotomy.
- Thus avoiding un-necessary delay in starting chemo therapy for patients with advanced disease.

STAGING :

AJCC TNM Staging system used.

T stage : (Fig. 2.2)

T1 : Tumour invades submucosa.

T2 : Tumour invades muscularis propria.

T3 : Tumour invades subserosal connective tissue without penetrating through serosa (visceral peritoneum) or invading adjacent structures.

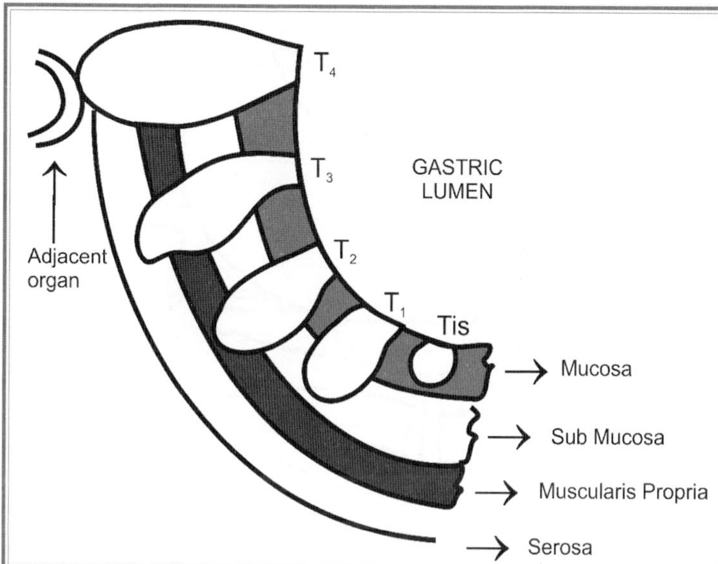

Fig. 2.2: TNM stage Ca ????

T4 : Tumour penetrating through serosa $\pm$ invading adjacent structures.

N stage :

N1 : Metastasis to 1-2 Lymph Nodes (LN).

N2 : Metastasis to 3-6 Lymph Nodes (LN).

N3 : Metastasis to >7 Lymph Nodes (LN).

M stage :

M0: No distant metastasis

M1: Distant metastasis present

Japanese Classification of Gastric Cancer:

They have described 16 LN stations **(Fig. 2.3)**

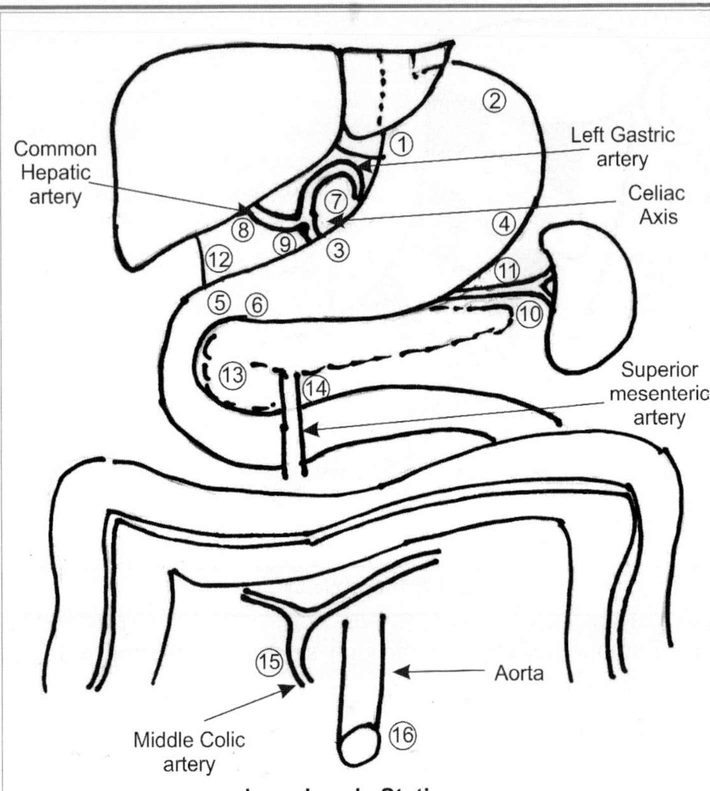

Fig. 2.3: Lymphnode Stations

1, 3, 5 : Along lesser curvature

2, 4, 6 : Along greater curvature

7 : Along Left Gastric artery

8 : Along Common Hepatic artery

9 : Celiac axis LN

10 : Splenic hilar LN

11 : Along Splenic artery

12 : Hepato-duodenal ligament LN

13 : Retro Pancreatic LN

14 : Along Superior Mesenteric vessels

15 : Along Middle Colic vessels

16 : Para-aortic LN

TERMINOLOGY specific to Ca Stomach :

- **Early Gastric Cancer** (described in detail later)**:**
  - It is defined as T1 disease with or without LN involvement (any N).

- **Low Risk Vs High Risk Disease :**
  - **Low Risk disease :**

    T1 or T2, N0 : Better survival

  - **High Risk disease :**

    T stage : > T2 *i.e.* T3, T4
N stage : > N0 *i.e.* N1 or higher } Poor survival with Increased unresectability

  - One of most important use of EUS is that it differentiates HIGH RISK from LOW RISK disease thus helping in prognostification.

TREATMENT :

Treatment Pathways are :

1) Surgery alone.
2) Neo Adjuvant Chemo Rx f/b surgery.
3) Chemo Rx alone.

Surgery :

- Status of Resection (R status) (By Hormanck).
  R0 → No residual disease → Good Long from survival.
  R1 → Microscopic residual disease.
  R2 → Gross residual disease.
- Surgery with RO resection remains Standard of care.
- **Distal gastric Ca :** D2 Sub total Gastrectomy with Bilroth II/Roux en Y Gastro-jejunostomy **(Fig. 2.4).**
- **Proximal gastric Ca :** D2 Total Gastrectomy with Roux en Y Esophago-jejunostomy **(Fig. 2.5).**
- Approach may be Open/Laparoscopic
- **Margin required : 6 cm**
- Atleast 15 Lymph nodes must be removed for satisfactory staging.
- **Levels of LN dissection :**
  D1 → Removal of stomach with perigastric nodes (LN stations: 1-6)
  D2 → D1 + celiac Axis clearance (LN station: 7,8,9,11) ± Splenic hilar LN clearance (station 10) ± Splenectomy
  D3 → D2 + Clearance of LN stations 12-14
  D4 → D3 + Clearance of LN stations 15, 16
- **Spleen preserving D2 resection is the recommended surgical approach**
- Adjuvant Chemo-Radiation indications :
  - T3, T4 tumours, Node positive,
  - R1/R2 resections

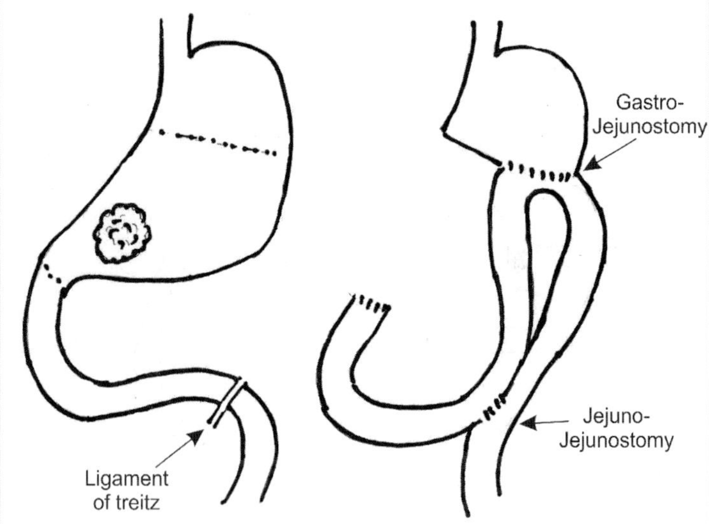

Fig. 2.4: Sub total Gastrectomy with Brauns Loop Gastro-jejunostomy

- Advanced tumours can be down staged with Neo Adj Chemo-Radiation :
  - Followed by Surgery
  - Followed by Adjuvant Chemotherapy
- Advanced tumours : Definitive Chemo-Radiation
- Chemotherapy agents :
  - ECF : Epirubicin, Cisplatin, 5-FU (MAGIC Trial)
  - DCF : Doxorubicin, Cisplatin, 5-FU
  - Newer drugs : Cetuximab
Transtuzumab

COMPLICATIONS in Ca stomach and its Treatment :

Bleeding : - Endoscopic hemostasis,

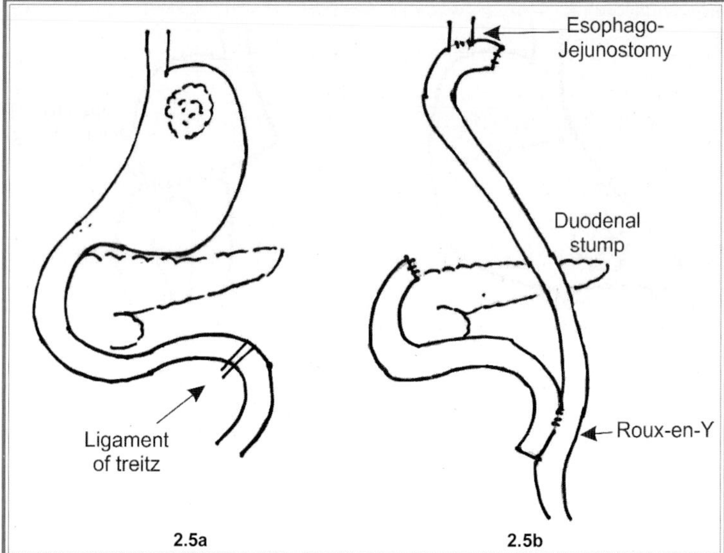

Fig. 2.5: Total Gastrectomy with Roux-en-Y any Esophago-Jejunostomy

- Angiography with Coil embolisation,
- Surgical resection.

Perforation : Biopsy and Primary closure/gastrectomy.

Obstruction :
- Dilation with stenting.
- Paliative Gastro-Jejunostomy.

Linitis Plastica : Its aggressive with high rate of complications.
Treatment : Total gastrectomy if symptomatic.

Survival after Surgery :

25-50% at 5 year.

Surveillance :

- 3-6 monthly in first 2 years,

- 6 monthly from third year onwards till 5 years
- History & Clinical Examination at all visits.
- Labs (CBC, LFT), Endoscopy and Imaging (X-ray chest and CT) as indicated

Special Mention:

A) SIEWERTS CLASSIFICATION for GE junction tumours :

Type I : Cancer associated with Barrett's or true esophageal Ca growing down to GE junction.

Type II : Tumour at true junction (within 2 cm of squamocolumnar junction).

Type III : Tumour of subcardial region.

B) EARLY GASTRIC CANCER :

- It is defined as T1 disease with or without LN involvement, (T1, any N).

- **DIAGNOSIS :**

1) Endoscopy based imaging technologies :

a) Chromoendoscopy :

- Subtle premalignant/early malignant lesions can be identified
- Can be used to ensure complete removal of neoplastic tissue after endoscopic excision

Special stains used :

i) Contrast stains : Indigo carmine – Pools into crypts

ii) Absorptive stains : Lugol's iodine – absorbed by glycogen

Methylene blue

iii) Reactive stains : Congo red – Red in alkaline pH
Black in acidic pH

b) Narrow band imaging :

- Uses only light with wavelength between 415 nm - 540 nm
- It facilitates enhanced visualisation of the vascular architecture of mucosa
- Altered vascular architecture suggests pathology

c) Endoscopic optical Coherence tomography :

- Principle same as B-mode USG, using infra-red light waves instead of acoustic waves.
- Provides High resolution, cross-sectional, tomographic images of microstructure of tissue.
- Real time imaging of multilayer architecture possible.
- Altered architecture suggests pathology.

Other Advances :

- Doppler optical Coherence tomography
- Spectroscopic optical Coherence tomography
- Ultra high resolution optical Coherence tomography

d) EUS : To evaluate depth of Ca invasion.

2) Serum markers :

a) Pepsinogen :
- I
- II

- Indicator of chief cell mass.
- Disproportionate fall in PG I compared to PG II suggests : Gastric Cancer.
- Very Low PG I values suggests an Advanced disease with Poor prognosis.
  - Can be used as SCREENING tool.

b) CA 72-4 and CEA :

Raised CA 72-4 is an indicator of advanced disease with dissemination.

3) Virtual Gastroscopy :

- Newer – Spasmolytic polypeptide levels
  Reduced E-Cadherin expression
  IL-IB gene polymorphism

- **TREATMENT options for Early Gastric Cancer :**
  - Endoscopic Mucosal Resection (EMR)
  - Endoscopic Submucosal dissection (ESD)

Criteria for endoscopic therapy :

- Limited to mucosa
- No ulcer
- < 2 cm in size
- No Lymphovascular invasion

If out of Criteria then :

- Minimally Invasive Resection Surgery

✡✡✡

Chapter 3

Colo-Rectal Carcinoma (CRC)

CANCER GENETICS

Fearon Vogelstein Model of Adenoma - Carcinoma Sequence :

Normal Epithelium

↓ Loss of APC (Initiation)

Dysplasia

(Abnormal crypt formation)

Earliest change

↓

Early Adenoma

↓ K Ras activation (Promotion)

Intermediate Adenoma

↓ Loss of DCC

Late Adenoma

↓ Loss of P53 (Late mutation)

Carcinoma

GENES INVOLVED :

1) Tumour supressor gene (Gatekeeper Gene) :

APC = Adenomatous Polyposis Coli gene : Chromosome 5

Loss of function

↓

Rise in Beta Cantenin levels

↓

WNT activation

↓

Rise in Cyclin D1 and MYC

↓

Cell proliferation

- APC : Mutation occurs early in Adenoma-Ca sequence with earliest pathological change being : Aberrant crypt foci
- APC : Germline Truncation mutation results in :

Familial Adenomatous Polyposis (FAP) :

- FAP : is Autosomal Dominant.
- Characterised by >100 almost thousand colorectal polyps by 20-30 years of age Some proceeding to Carcinoma.
- Account for <1% cases of all CRC.
- Average age for adenoma formation is 15 Years.
- CRC develops in nearly 100% by age of 40.
- Types of FAP :
    1) Classic FAP : Mutation between Codon 1250 & codon 1464.

2) Mutation close to 5' end : Attenuated FAP with less polyp (< 100) & Rectal sparing.
3) Mutation close to 3' end : even more attenuated form, rare.

- **SYNDROMES associated with FAP :**

➢ ***Gardner Syndrome :***

FAP with :

- Osteoma
- Dermoid tumor
- Desmoid tumor

So also :

- CHRPE : Congenital hypertrophy of retinal pigment epithelium
- Medulloblastoma
- Fundic gastric polyp
- Peri ampullary Cancer
- Thyroid papillary Cancer

- The extra intestinal manifestation depends on location of mutation on the gene
- M/C malignancy after CRC & M/C cause of death after CRC is eliminated by surgery : Peri ampulary Cancer.
- **Spigelmans criteria** used to predict malignant risk of duodenal polyposis

➢ ***Turcots Syndrome :***

FAP with Brain tumours (M/C : Medulloblastoma)

Autosomal ressesive

- **DIAGNOSIS :**

  Protein Truncation test } genetic testing
  Direct DNA sequencing }

- **SCREENING :**

  Annual colonoscopy beginning 10-12 years of age.

- **TREATMENT :**

  - Prophylactic surgery:

    Total Procto-Colectomy with ileal pouch anal anastomosis (IPAA).

Special mention : **MYH Associated Polyposis**

- MYH is a DNA damage repair gene.
- Therefore when mutated it promotes APC damage.
- MYH mutation results in a FAP like Phenotype without characteristic germline APC mutation.
- Autosomal Recessive, therefore heterozygous individuals not afflicted & off springs also spared unless spouse is also a carrier.
- Siblings however may be affected.

Other Tumour suppressor genes:

- **P53, DCC, SMAD4**
- **P53 – guardian of genome** (Chromosome 17)

  Mutation occurs late in Adenoma-Ca sequence.

2) **Mismatch Repair gives (MMR) (care taker genes) :**

   - They Correct DNA Replication errors.
   - Include : MSH, MLH, PMS.

- Mutation → Produce microsatellite instability (MSI).
- Results in Hereditary non polyposis colon cancer (HNPCC)

Hereditary non polyposis colon cancer :

- MMR genes are located on chromosome 2, 3 & 7.
- Responsible for 3-5% of all CRC.
- In them incidence of adenoma and CRC is similar to general population.
- However the adenoma develop at a younger age & have higher incidence of high grade dysplasia and villous architecture.
- The CRC that develops are usually poorly differentiated with signet ring histology with "crohns like pattern of infiltrating lymphocytes".
- Increased incidence of synchronous/metachronous Ca.

• **TYPES :**

- Lynch syndrome I : CRC only
- Lynch syndrome II : CRC + [***Endometrial Ca (M/C), gastric cancer, ovarian cancer, Urinary tract cancers***, pancreatic cancers, thyroid cancers, CNS tumours (Glioblastoma)]
- Muir Torre Syndrome = HNPCC + tumours of sebaceous glands + keratocanthomas

• **DIAGNOSIS :**

- Genetic testing for : - MSH2, MLH1
  - MSI testing

- **Revised Amsterdam's criteria :** To identify at risk patients for genetic testing
    1. 3 or more relative diagnosed with HNPCC associated malignancy, one being first degree relative of the other 2
    2. 2 successive generations affected
    3. 1 or more case being diagnosed before 50 years
    4. FAP excluded
- **Bethesda guidelines** used to direct patient selection for MSI testing

- **SCREENING protocol in HNPCC :**

  Prevention better than cure

  - Colonoscopy every 1-2 years beginning at 20-25 years or 10 years before the earliest diagnosis of CRC in family, whichever comes first.
  - Transvaginal USG, endometrial biopsy & CA-125 testing annually starting at 25-35 years.
  - Annual abdominal USG & urinary cytology starting at 25 years (for urinary tract Ca).
  - Upper GI scopy starting at 35 years.

3) Oncogene :

- Mutation in oncogenes are "gain in function" mutations.
- Whereas mutation in tumour suppressor genes are "loss in function" mutations.
- **K-ras** oncogene mutation causes tumour promotion in intermediate polyp

Oncogenes produce :

- Growth factor : TGF beta, EGF.
- Receptors.
- Signal transducers.

Colorectal Polyp

Polyp is any mass projecting into the lumen.

Above surface of intestinal epithelium.

ADENOMATOUS POLYP :

Pathology :

- Grossly (**Fig. 3.1**) — Pedunculated / Sessile

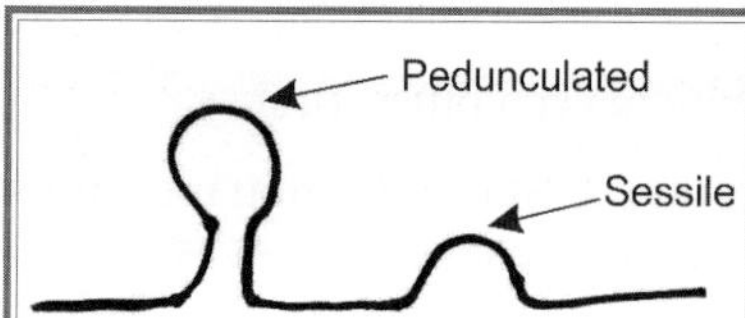

Fig. 3.1: Types of Polyp

- Microscopy : (**Fig. 3.2**)
  - Tubular
  - Villous
  - Tubulovillous

- Most common : tubular > tubulo-villous > villous
- Tubular : Tend to be pedunculated with less atypia
- Villous : Tend to be Sessile with severe atypia
- Polyps at High risk for malignacy → villous polyps, sessile polyps

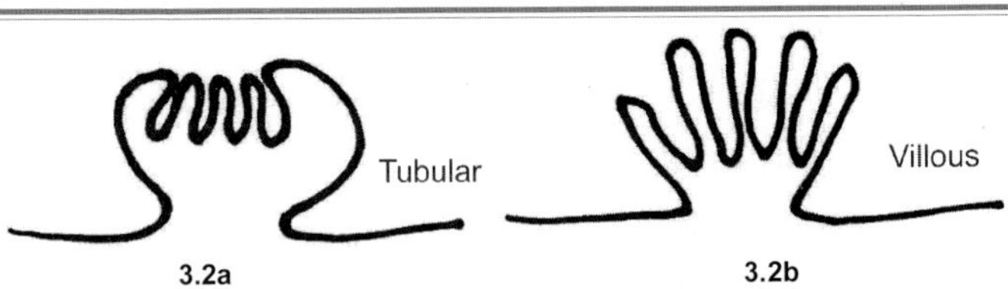

Fig. 3.2: Tubular Vs Villous Polyp

- ↳ Size > 2 cm : 50% chance of Ca
- ↳ Size < 1 cm : less than 5% chance

- ➢ Treatment is polypectomy, serving dual purpose, providing tissue for histopathology and resulting in possible cure
- ➢ Pedunculated polyp : Colonscopic Snare polypectomy
- ➢ Sessile polyp : Segmental colectomy preferred though EMR can be done for small polyps
- ➢ A polyp may harbour foci of cancer which may be carcinoma in situ or invasive carcinoma.
  - ↳ Carcinoma in situ (limited to mucosa by muscularis mucosa) does not metastasize & complete excision is adequate treatment.
  - ↳ A polyp is said to contain invasive Ca when Muscularis Mucosa is breached.
  - ↳ If invasive, classified as per **Haggitts Classification** based on depth of invasion **(Fig. 3.3)**

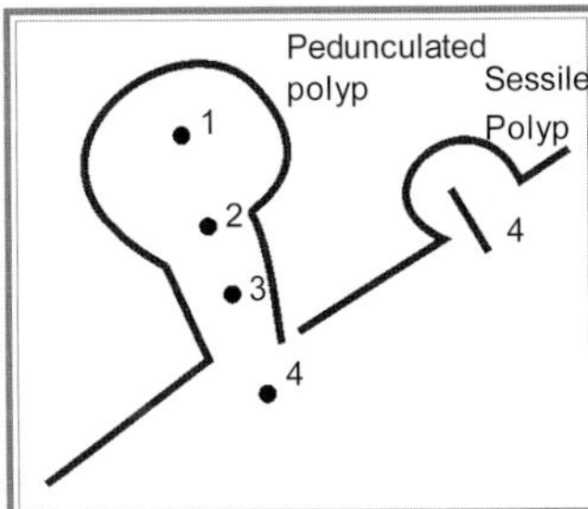

Fig. 3.3: Haggitts Classification

Cis – 0
Head – I
Neck – II
Stalk – III
Bowel wall – IV

- Invasive Ca in sessile polyp is always grade IV
- Treatment of polyp with foci of cancer as per Haggitts class:
  - Level 1, 2, 3 → Low possibility of LN invasion, hence colonoscopic polypectomy may suffice if margin is free
  - Level 4 → 10% chance of LN invasion, hence requires aggressive treatment i.e. Surgical resection

Other colorectal polyps :

- Hyperplastic polyp : HPR = saw toothed/serrated
- Mucus retention polyp
- Hamartomatous polyp
- Inflammatory polyp

Colorectal Carcinoma

- Very common cancer worldwide.
- 3rd most common cancer in USA.
- Less prevalent in India although incidence is rising.

ETIOLOGY :

- Adenomatous Polyp :

  Higher risk with : Villous > tubular polyp

Sessile > Pedunculated polyp

Polyp > 1 cm

Arising as per adenoma – Ca sequence (described previously)

- Dietary & lifestyle factors :
  - ➢ Westernised diet
  - ➢ High in fat, low in fibre with low fruit intake
- Inflammatory bowel disease.
  Ulcerative Colitis > Crohns disease.
- Genetic/Hereditary Cancers, *e.g :* FAP, HNPCC.
- Smoking & alcohol.
- Personal history of cancers at other sites : breast, thyroid, ovary.
- Family history of cancer in colo-rectum or at other sites : breast, thyroid, ovary.
- Asbestos.
- Increased risk after cholecystectomy as there is increased exposure of bile to right colon (controversial).
- Streptococcus Bovis bacteraemia.
- Ureterosigmoidostomy.
- Pelvic irradiation.

Protective: Diet high in fibre, calcium, Vit D, selenium, hormone replacement therapy & Aspirin reduces risk.

HISTOLOGY :

- 98% are Adenocarcinoma.

Others :
- Carcinoid found more around caecum & rectum.
- Lymphoma found more around caecum.

LOCATION :

- Most common in rectum (20%), followed by: Sigmoid colon > Caecum > Transverse colon > Ascending colon > Descending colon > Splenic flexure > Hepatic flexure.
- $2/3^{rd}$ in left colon, $1/3^{rd}$ in right colon.
- M/C site of distant mets : liver > lung.

FORMS :

It occurs in either of the three forms : Sporadic, Hereditary or Familial

1) **Hereditary :** Characterised by family History, young age at onset with other specific defects.

2) **Familial (new concept) :**
   - Increased lifetime risk for members of family with index patient developing cancer < 50 years of age.
   - Risk increases with increasing number of affected family members.

3) **Sporadic :** M/C form

   Absence of family history with cancer developing at older age and Mutation Limited to tumor.

SIGNS/SYMPTOMS :

Colonic :

Lt sided Ca: are usually constricting/stricturing causing gradual obstruction resulting in a change in bowel habits with increasing constipation.

Rt sided Ca: rarely cause obstruction in early stages due to wide luminal size. They usually cause malena, anaemia, fatigue, pain, mass.

Bleeding : Haematochezia more common with left sided tumours and malena more common with right sided ones.

Anemia : Any male/non-menstruating female with Anaemia : Do a colonoscopy rule out Ca.

Sigmoid Ca may mimic diverticulitis, may even cause colo-vesical, colo-vaginal fistula.

Rectal :

- Hematochezia is the most common presenting symptom.
- Tenesmus : Sense of incomplete defecation with the sensation that there is more faeces to be passed.
- Spurious diarrhoea : Patient may attempt to empty the rectum several times a day with passage of some flatus and some bloody slime.
- Early morning bloody Diarrhea.
- Annular obstructing Ca: Increasing constipation progressing to obstruction.

DIFERENTIAL DIAGNOSIS:

UC, CD, Radiation proctitis, procidentia, solitary rectal ulcer.

Colitis cystica profunda.

WORK UP :

- History + examination
- CBC, LFT
- Serum CEA levels : Tumour Marker

IMAGING :

- X-ray Chest : to rule out pulmonary metastsis

- CECT with rectal contrast
- MRI
- PET-CT

} loco regional staging & rule out metastasis

ENDOSCOPY :

- Colonoscopy : Describes Site, extent, nature & provides tissue for Biopsy.

  To rule out synchronous polyp/Ca.

- EUS : Helps in T and N staging.

ADDITIONAL INVESTIGATION FOR RECTAL CA :

- Pelvic CT,
- Endorectal coil MRI : best for overall staging
- EUS : best for T staging

STAGING :

AJCC TNM Staging system used.

T stage :

T1 : Tumour invades submucosa

T2 : Tumour invades muscularis propria

T3 : Tumour invades subserosal connective tissue without penetrating through serosa (visceral peritoneum) or invading adjacent structures

T4 : Tumour penetrating through serosa +/- invading adjacent structures

N stage :

N1 : Metastasis to 1-3 LNs

N2 : Metastasis to 4 or more LNs

M stage :

M0: No distant metastasis

M1: Distant metastasis present

STAGE :

Stage I : T1, T2

Stage II : T3, T4

Stage III : N1, N2

Stage IV : M1

Modified DUKE's Staging :

A : Confined to mucosa

B1 : Partially penetrating the muscularis propria } modified by Kirklin

B2 : Fully penetrating the muscularis propria } modified by Kirklin

C1 : Spread to 1-4 LNs } Modified by Astler-Coller

C2 : Spread to more than 4 LNs } Modified by Astler-Coller

D : Distant metastasis ⟶ modified by Turnbull

Pathological staging	vs	**Clinical staging**
• Done Post-op		• Done Pre-op
• Determines need for post-op Adjuvant Rx		• Determines need for pre-op Neo-Adj therapy

PROGNOSIS :

Prognostic Factors :

- Most important : Stage
- Single most important independent factor : LN status

Others :

1) KRAS mutation → EGF-R inhibitors like cetuximab & panitumumab cannot be given in patients with K-ras mutation positivity.
2) Serum CEA levels.
3) Number of satellite tumor deposits.
4) Tumor regression grade.
5) MSI : Micro satellite instability.
6) PNI : Perineural invasion.
7) CRM : Circumferential resection margin.

TREATMENT of Colonic Ca :

Surgical resection whenever possible is the treatment of choice

OBJECTIVE :

Removal of primary Ca with adequate margins with resection of lymphatics which parallel arterial supply to greatest extent possible & restoration of G-I continuity

SURGERY :

- **For tumours involving caecum, ascending colon, hepatic flexure :**

  Right Hemicolectomy (Fig. 3.4) it includes resection of atleast 6 cm of terminal ileum upto part of transverse colon supplied by right branch of middle colic artery

- **Transverse colon lesions :**

  Extended right hemicolectomy with Ileo-Descending Anastomosis : right hemicolectomy plus resection of whole of transverse colon along with splenic flexure **(Fig. 3.5).**

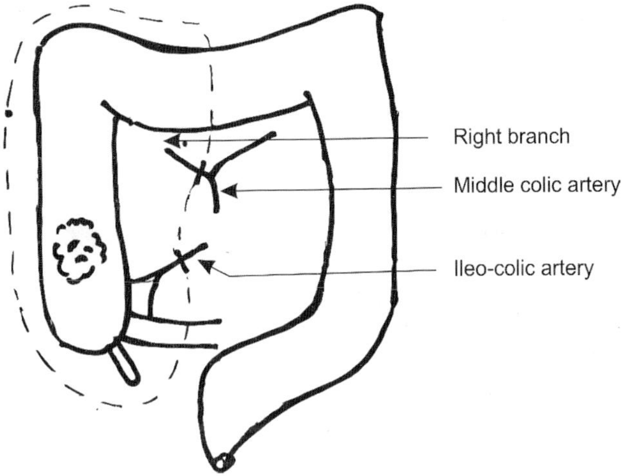

Fig. 3.4: Right Hemicolectomy

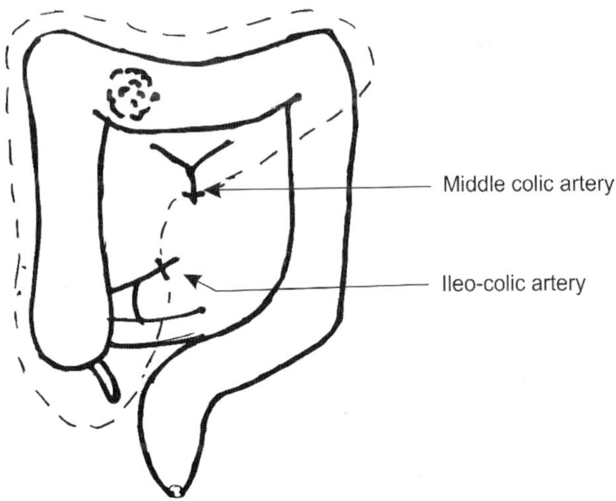

Fig. 3.5: Extended right hemicolectomy with Ileo-Descending Anastomosis

Or

Transverse colectomy : Resection of transverse colon (middle colic territory) **(Fig. 3.6).**

- **Descending colon lesions :**
  Left hemi colectomy with colorectal anastomosis **(Fig. 3.7).**
- **Sigmoid Ca :**
  Sigmoidectomy or High Anterior resection (Fig. 3.8).

STAGE WISE TREATMENT :

Stage I :

Surgery followed by active surveillance :

- Surveillance should be intensive, especially in the first 2 years.
- Goal of surveillance is close follow-up to detect recurrence at an early stage, amenable to treatment.

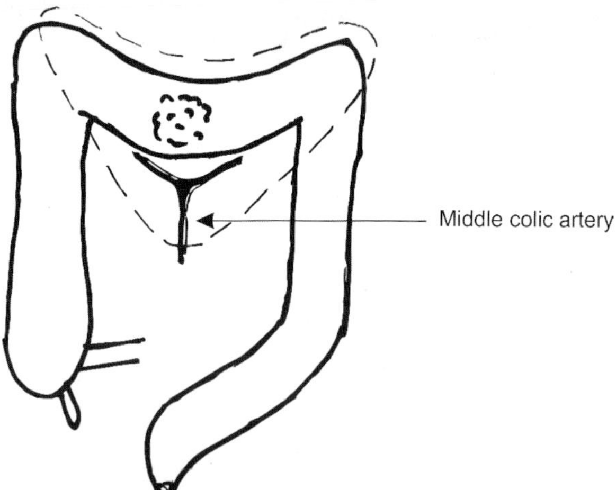

Fig. 3.6: Transverse colectomy

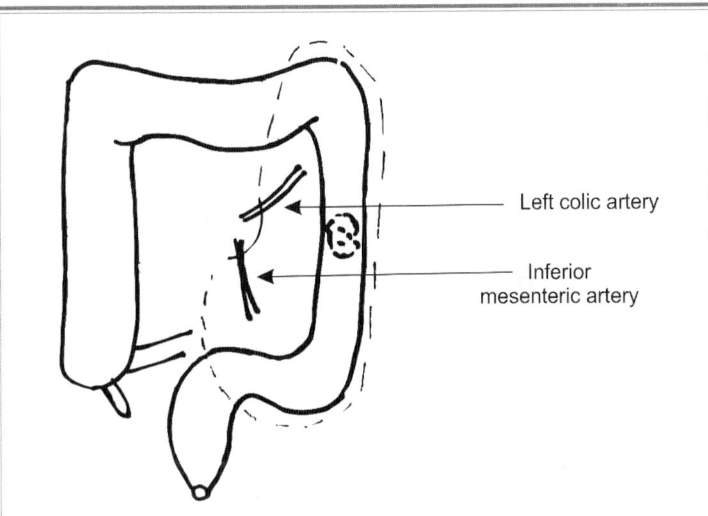

Fig. 3.7: Left hemi colectomy with colorectal anastomosis

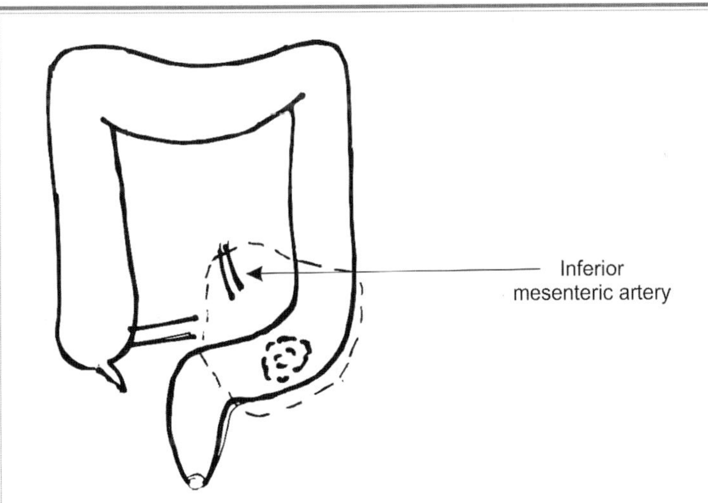

Fig. 3.8: Sigmoidectomy or High Anterior resection

- It includes:
  - Annual colonoscopy
  - 3 monthly CEA for 1st 2 years
  - if rising → CT, MRI, & PET apart from colonoscopy.

Stage II :

- Surgery followed by adjuvant chemotherapy followed by surveillance
- Chemotherapy Regimen commonly advocated: FolFOx, it includes:
  Follinic Acid + 5-FU + Oxaliplatin
- Indication:
  - T4 tumours
  - <12 LNs Sampled
  - Grade 3/4 tumours
  - Perforation
- 6 cycles given over 12 weeks with 2 weeks gap in between each cycle

Cycle :

Day 1: - 80 mg oxaliplatin in 1 pint 5% dextrose

- 200 mg Leucovorin in 1 pint 5% dextrose
- Together over 2 hours through Y channel
- followed by: Bolus 5-FU 400 mg
- followed by: 5 FU infusion 600 mg over 22 hours

Day 2: Only leucovorin and 5FU

- CBC & RFT is done in between each cycle.
- Inj. Filgrastrin/Neupogen if Leucopenia detected (300 mg x 3 days).

Stage III :

- Surgery & Adj chemo therapy } FolFOx
  Or
  fol FIri (Follinic acid + 5FU + Inrinotecan)
- followed by Surveillance.

Stage IV :

- Definitive Chemo therapy → Main stay of treatment
- Surgical resection for palliation.

New agents being tried :

- EGRF inhibitor → Cetuximab, Panitumumab, Bevacizumab.
  KRAS testing recommended prior to their use.

TREATMENT for Rectal Ca :

Cons :

- The retroperitoneal location of the rectum in a narrow pelvis with proximity to urogenital structures, autonomic Nerves & anal sphincters makes Surgery difficult.
- Dissection medial to Endo-pelvic fascia investing the mesorectum → leads to recurrence
- Dissection lateral to it → results in Autonomic nerve damage - Impotence/Bladder Dysfunction

Pros :

- Distance from small bowels allows radiation

Prior to treatment planning, Tumor has to be characterised, as to its →

- Distance from Anal verge

- Extent
- Invasion (T & N stage)

Multimodality therapy is usually required

STAGE WISE TREATMENT :

Stage I : Local excision or radical resection depending on tumour factors

Stage II : Pre-op chemo radiation f/b radical resection

Stage III : Pre-op chemo radiation f/b radical resection

Stage IV : Palliation

NeoAdjuvant Therapy

- Pre-op therapy given to down stage the tumour.
- Recommended in Stage II & III tumours.
- It may be either :
    - **Short course** Radio therapy : 25 CGY over 5 days
      OR
    - **Long course** Chemo-Radio therapy
      Radiation 4500 CGY + Fol FOx over 6 week followed by wait for 6 week followed by Surgery.

SURGERY FOR RECTAL CA :

1) **Local Excisions :**

for mobile tumour
- < 4 cm in size
- involving < 40% of circumference
- < 6 cm from Anal Verge
- **T1**
- G1/G2

- With no lymphatic OR vascular invasion

- It involves : Excision of full thickness of rectal wall involved by the tumor with Adequate margin.
- No LN removal possible.
- High chance of Recurrence.
- Can be used for palliation in Advanced disease/Old frail patient.

Newer Approach : **Transanal Endoscopic microscopic surgery (TEMS)**

- It includes use of a specially designed proctoscope 4 cm wide with 4 functional ports for :
  - CO_2 inflation
  - Suction
  - Water irrigation
  - Pressure monitoring
- ***Advantage*** ***:*** Excellent exposure
- ***Disadvantage :***
  - Expensive
  - high learning curve
  - amenable only for a few Lesions
- Closure of defect is not necessary as it is below the peritoneal Reflection.

- ***Complication :***
  - Bleeding
  - Perforation which fecal soilage

- Fecal incontinence
- Urinary incontinence

2) **Fulguration :** For symptomatic relief in old frail patients/ Advanced disease

3) **Anterior Resection (AR) :**

- For tumours located more than 5 cm above the anal verge
- Sphincter saving surgery
- Laproscopic approach preferred over open
- Based on the relation of the distal resection margin to the peritoneal reflection and levator ani surgery may be classified as:
  - Above peritoneal reflection: Anterior resction (AR) (called as High AR by some)
  - Below peritoneal reflection: Low AR
  - At level of levator ani: Ultra-low AR
- Descending colon anastomosed to rectal stump
- Recently interspincteric resection with colo-anal anastomosis are being performed for very low rectal cancers located 3 cm above the anal verge
- Concept of **Total Mesorectal Excision (TME)** must be followed in order to achieve negative circumferential resection margin (CRM) which is associated with decreased local recurrence rates and improved long term survival.
- Proximal resection margin required: 5 cm
- Distal rectal resection margin required: 2 cm
- Suggested distal mesorectal margin: 5cm

- **Anterior Resection Syndrome (ARS)**: Fecal urgency, frequent bowel movements & incontinence that occurs after AR. Lower the colo-rectal anastomosis, higher the risk of ARS. Usually settles with conservative management with diet modification.

4) **Abdomino-perineal resection (APR)** = Miles procedure
   - Concomitant abdominal and perineal dissection resulting in complete excision of rectum and anus
   - For lower rectal tumours < 5 cm from anal verge
   - Permanent colostomy created
   - Concept of TME must be followed to decrease local recurrence and improve long term survival

5) **Spincter sparring APR:** Said to be associated with better perineal wound healing

FOR PATIENTS PRESENTING WITH COMPLETE INTESTINAL OBSTRUCTION

↓

Water-soluble contrast Enema → Diagnosis; Anatomic level of obstruction

↓

Surgery

- **Surgery for obstructing Ca :**
  - **Right sided colonic obstruction:** Right hemicolectomy with ileo-transverse Anastomosis.
  - **Descending or Sigmoid colon:**

    Hartmann Surgery : left colonic resection with descending colostomy with closure of rectal stump

OR

- Left colonic resection with on table Lavage (through Appendix/ileum) followed by primary colo-rectal Anastomosis

OR

- Subtotal colectomy which ileo-rectal Anastomosis

- **Rectal obstruction:**

  Loop colostomy followed by neo adjuvant CRT with resection of primary later.

- **Newer treat modality:**

  Endoscopic stenting & resuscitation followed by complete workup & elective resection.

SCREENING for CRC :

After 50 years.

- Faecal occult blood testing annually & Flexible Sigmoidoscopy every 5 years starting at 50 years.

Or

- Better option : Total colonic examination (Colonoscopy or Double contrast barium enema) every 10 years starting at 50 years.
- Colonoscopy superior to Double contrast barium enema.
- The latter is usually only performed if colonoscopy is contraindicated or not available.

✡✡✡

Chapter 4

Carcinoma Anal Canal & Anal Margin

- M/C type of CA anal canal: Squamous Cell Ca> Basal Cell Ca >Melanoma
- Median age at diagnosis : 60 years
- M/C site of metastasis : Lung
- M/C site of LN metastasis : Inguinal LNs
- Epidermoid carcinoma of the anus includes SCC, cloacogenic carcinoma, transitional carcinoma and basaloid carcinoma. The clinical behavior and natural history of these tumors are similar

ETIOLOGY :

1. HPV infection : 16, 18, 31, 33
2. HIV or immunosuppression
3. Smoking
4. Anal receptive intercourse
5. Sexual promiscuity
6. Chronic inflammation
7. History of vulvar or cervical cancer in females.

Precursor lesion : Anal intra-epithelial neoplasia.

SIGNS/SYMPTOMS :

- Most patients present with bleeding and pain
- M/C symptom : Bleeding PR
- Patients are frequently misdiagnosed as having a benign anorectal condition such as hemorrhoids

- Symptoms suggestive of advanced disease : Incontinence, change in bowel habits, pelvic pain, rectovaginal or rectovesical fistulas usually a/w infiltration into the sphincters or penetration into the rectal wall

DIAGNOSIS :

- Proctoscopy with biopsy : Investigation of choice for diagnosis of anal canal tumours
- CT abdomen and pelvis : Helps in locoregional staging
  To evaluate distant metastasis

STAGING :

AJCC TNM staging system used for anal canal & anal margin tumours

Tis : Carcinoma in situ (Bowen disease, high-grade squamous, intraepithelial lesions (HSIL), anal intraepithelial neoplasia II-III (AINII-III).

T1 : Tumour < 2 cm in size

T2 : > 2 cm but < 5 cm in size

T3 : > 5 cm in size

T4 (Anal Canal) : Invading adjacent structures : vagina, urethra, or bladder (involvement of the sphincter muscle alone, rectal wall, or perirectal subcutaneous tissue or skin is not classified as T4).

T4 (Anal Margin) : Invading deep into extra dermal structure : skeletal muscle or bone.

N1 : Metastases to perirectal LNs.

N2 : Metastases to unilateral internal iliac and/or inguinal LNs.

N3 : Metastases to perirectal and/or bilateral internal iliac and/ or bilateral inguinal LNs.

M1: Distant metastasis

TREATMENT :

- Treatment of choice for anal canal Ca : NIGRO regimen (Chemoradiation)
- More than 80% cases can be cured by chemoradiation.
- APR for any residual tumor left behind after chemoradiation
- Chemotherapy : 5-FU + Mitomycin C or Cisplatin.
- Radiation : 30 Gy
- First chemotherapy is given followed by radiotherapy

PROGNOSIS :

- Overall 5-year survival : 66%

Anal Margin Tumours

- These tumours arise on the perianal skin beyond the anal verge.
- Metastases are late and rare, and recurrences are typically locoregional.
- Symptoms include pain, bleeding, itching, and palpable mass.
- Diagnosis is often suspected by the experienced clinician on inspection, but biopsy prior to definitive treatment is imperative.

- Squamous cell carcinoma of the anal margin is treated by primary surgical excision similar to skin cancers.
- Small lesion : Wide-local excision.
- Large lesion or sphincter involvement : Chemoradiation followed by surgery for residual disease.

✡✡✡

Chapter 5

Gastro-intestinal Carcinoid Tumour

- Arise from Enterochomaffin cells/Kulchitsky cells/ Argentaffin cells in crypts of lieberkuhn of GI tract.
- Contain multipotent cells which are capable of secreting a wide variety of humoral products.
- Stain with silver compounds.
- Arise most commonly from GIT (M/C) & Respiratory tract.
- Distribution : Bronchus > ileum > rectum > appendix > colon > stomach (pneumonic = BIRACS).
- Most commonly in 5th decade.
- **20% multicentric** (highest for any GI malignancy).
- There is usually a frequent co-existence of another GI malignancy (M/C colorectal Ca).
- Associated with MEN 1.

- **Primary concern** → Malignant potential

  ↓

  Hepatic metastasis

  ↓

  Carcinoid Syndrome

- Malignant potential based on :

  Site : ileal > Appendicial

  Size : < 1 cm : very low

  > 1 cm : risk increases drastically.

CLASSIFICATION :

Classified according to embryologic site of origin and secretory products.

- **Foregut :** Respiratory tract, thymus, stomach, proximal duodenum

  Secrete : Low levels of serotonin

  High levels of 5-Hydroxytryptophan, ACTH

- **Midgut :** Small intestine, Right colon, Appendix

  Secrete : High level of serotonin

- **Hindgut :** Distal colon & Rectum

  Secrete : Low level of serotonin

  High level of Somatostatin, Peptide YY

- Others products : Histamine, dopamine, prostaglandins (PG) substance P.
- Of most importance Serotonin & substance P

PATHOLOGY :

Grossly :

- They usually present as a submucosal nodule which is yellowish on cut section
- They may be associated with large mesenteric mass due to LN's & Intense desmoplastic reaction.
- Very slow growth, but once serosa breached.

  ↓

  Intense desmoplastic reaction

  ↓

  Kinking of bowel

  ↓

Obstruction
↓
Venous then arterial compromise → ischemia

SIGNS & SYMPTOMS :

- Majority asymptomatic.
- Symptoms usually results from intermittent sub acute intestinal obstruction resulting from intussusceptions or LN mass & mesenteric desmoplasia causing kinking

Carcinoid Syndrome :

- Seen in less than < 10% of carcinoids.
- Usually seen in small intestinal carcinoids with extensive hepatic metastasis.

  Or

  Extra intestinal carcinoids → Respiratory tract, Ovary, testes, retro peritoneum
- It occurs due to : Evasion of 1st pass metabolism of humoral agents in liver, resulting in their raised blood levels.
- Mainly due to Serotonin, Histamine, Substance P.

- **Symptoms of Carcinoid syndrome:**
  - **Vasomotor** → Cutaneous flushing, Types:
    1) Diffuse erythematous flushing (short lived).
    2) Violaceous flushing is similar to Diffuse erythematous flushing but attacks last longer.

       Some develop permanent cyanotic flush.
    3) Prolonged flushes, lasting 2-3 days.
    4) Bright red patchy flushing, seen in Gastric carcinoid

➢ **GIT** → Secretory diarrhoea

Explosive, watery diarrhoea

Due to serotonin

Therapy :

- Methylsurgide → causes retroperitoneal fibrosis → hence no longer used
- Ondansetron
- Ketanserin
- Cypro heptadine

➢ **CVS** → Right sided valvular disease

pulmonary stenosis > tricuspid insufficiency > tricuspid stenosis > pulmonary insufficiency.

➢ **RS** → Asthmatic Attacks

➢ Excessive diversion of dietary tryptophan leads to **Pellegra**: Diarrhoea, dementia & dermatitis.

DIAGNOSIS :

- **Blood tests :**

  ➢ 24 hr urinary 5-HIAA levels.

  (5-Hydroxy indole acetic Acid),

  +

  Serum chromogranin A levels.

  ➢ Serum chromogranin A levels also used for surveillance after surgery.

  Increased levels correlates with poor prognosis.

- **Provocative testing with pentagastrin:** stimulating symptoms.

- **BMFT :** Multiple filling defects due to fibrosis & kinking
- **CT:** Investigation of choice for detecting lymphatic & hematogenous metastasis & Mesenteric disease

LOCALISATION :

- Somatostatin receptor scan using 111 Indium labelled Pentetreotide : Investigation of choice for localisation.
- CT
- MRI
- PET : not of proven benefit

TREATMENT :

Small intestinal carcinoids :

< 1 cm without LN invasion	: segmental resection
> 1 cm, LN invasion, multiple tumor	: wide excision of bowel & mesentery

Terminal ileal → right hemicolectomy.

Duodenal : Excision if feasible, or else Whipple PD.

- At surgery, Check for multicentric disease
- Even in Advanced disease with extensive mesentric involvement :

  Surgical debulking has a role as it provides durable palliation
- hepatic mets → Metastatectomy

  if it recurs : Chemo/Radio Embolisation
- During Anaesthesia → Chance of carcinoid crisis is always present, with Hypotension, flushing, bronchospasm and Arrythmia occuring

  Therapy includes : IV Hydrocortisone, IV octreotide, IV Anti histamine

Medical treatment :

- Octreotide
- 2nd generation drugs → pasireotide
- IFN-α
- Antisecretory drugs :
  - Methylsurgide → Causes retroperitoneal fibrosis → no longer used
  - Ondansetron
  - Ketanserin
  - Cypro heptadine
- Chemo therapy in cases unresponsive to other modality OR with high proliferation rate.
  - Otherwise not of any benefit because of slow growth rate

    It includes : Streptozocin + 5 FU/Cyclophosphamide

    Or

    DEF = dacarbazine + epirubicin + 5-FU

Targeted Therapy :

- Bevacizumab
- Sunitinib/Sorafenib
- Everolimus

Most promising newer therapy : Targeted radiotherapy (Smart bombs) using radio labelled stomatostatin Analogue

Prognosis :

Best compared to other intestinal Ca.

✡✡✡

Chapter 6

Gastro-intestinal Lymphoma

- Tumour of Lymphatic origin.
- They may be classified as Hodgkin's lymphoma and non-Hodgkin's lymphoma.

Hodgkin's lymphoma →

- Arising from B lymphocytes
- Reed Sternberg cells are the tumour cells

Types :

1. Nodular sclerosis
2. Mixed
3. Lymphocytic Rich/Predominant
4. Lymphocyte depleted
5. Unclassified

- Spreads from one Lymph node to another in systematic manner with constitutional Symptoms.

Ann Arbor Staging :

I : One LN group involved

II : 2 or more LN groups on same side of diaphragm involved

III : Involvement of Lymphatics on either side of diaphragm

IV : Extra Lymphatic spread

GI Lymphoma :

- Majority of Gastro-intestinal lymphomas are of Non Hodgkin's type.

Gastrointestinal Lymphoma

- Non-Hodgkin's lymphomas may be divided into nodal and extranodal lymphoma.
- The gastrointestinal tract is the most common site of extranodal lymphoma.
- Most common site is Stomach > small intestine > colo-rectum.
- M/C site in stomach : Antrum.
- Rectal lymphoma is the rarest of all primary gastrointestinal lymphomas.
- It is M/C. Non-epithelial tumour of GI tract.
- Constitute 20% of all lymphoma.

DEFINITION :

Dawson *et al* established criteria for the diagnosis of primary gastrointestinal lymphoma.

These are :

1) The absence of clinically enlarged lymph nodes on physical examination,
2) The absence of enlarged mediastinal lymph nodes on chest radiograph,
3) Normal hematologic laboratory values and bone marrow biopsy, and
4) Normal-appearing liver and spleen,

All in the setting of lymphoma occurring in a portion of the gastrointestinal tract

In the current era of CT, the criteria has been expanded to include the exclusion of retroperitoneal or mediastinal lymphadenopathy.

ETIOLOGY :

- H. Pylori → Strongly associated with gastric MALToma. Other organisms linked :
  - Campylobacter jejuni
  - HTLV
  - EBV
- Immuno-supression due to :
  - HIV
  - Post-transplant Immuno-suppression
- Celiac sprue/Enteropathy associated with T cell Lymphoma
- IBD : inflammatory bowel disease
- Genetic predisposition

PATHOLOGY :

WHO Classification :

1) Diffuse Large B cell Lymphoma (DLBC) (M/C)* 55%
2) Extra nodal marginal Lymphoma (MALToma) (2nd M/C) 40%
3) Follicular cell Lymphoma }
4) Mantle cell Lymphoma } rare
5) Burkitts Lymphoma }

STAGING :

Ann Arbor staging system is widely used

IE : Confirmed to GI tract

IIE : Spread to regional LN

IIIE : Spread to other intra-abdominal organs

IVE : Beyond Abdomen to chest, bone marrow

Gastric Lymphoma

- 60-70 years
- M>F
- M/C site for GI lymphoma
- M/C site : Antrum

ETIOLOGY : (Discussed previously)

PATHOLOGY :

DLBC lymphoma :

- M/C histologic subtype is diffuse large B-cell lymphoma.
- Generally aggressive.
- Generally arise de novo as a primary lesion but may occasionally occur from progression of :
    - ➢ CLL – SLL, Follicular Lymphoma, MALToma.

MALToma :

- Second most common is MALT-associated B-cell lymphoma.
- These are low-grade tumors.
- It is often preceded by a chronic Helicobacter pylori infection & can be successfully treated by H. pylori eradication alone.
- Characteristic genetic abnormality : t(11 :18) which increases nuclear factor KB activity & impairs apoptotic signalling.
- t(11:18) & BCL-10 nuclear expression predict non responsiveness to H. Pylori eradication.

Burkitts Lymphoma :

- Aggressive, rare, associated with EBV
- Involves cardia/Body of stomach
- Three clinical forms :
    1. Endemic : in children, in Africa
    2. Sporadic : no geographic predilection,
    3. Immunodeficiency-associated : HIV, transplant, congenital

SIGNS/SYMPTOMS :

- Epigastric pain, early satiety.
- Fatigue.
- Overt bleeding is uncommon but **Anaemia** is very common.
- Constitutional symptoms are rare.

DIAGNOSIS :

1) OGD scopy :
    - Describes Site, extent, nature & provides tissue for Biopsy
    - At times it may show non-specific gastritis.
    - Biopsy may be non-diagnostic because of sub mucosal spread rather than mucosal involvement

2) EUS : identifies
    - ➢ Depth of penetration
    - ➢ Perivisceral LN status

3) H. Pylori testing :

    Non-invasive : - Urea Breath test, Serology

    Invasive : - CLO test : rapid urease test (RUT)
    - Pathology
    - Culture

STAGING : done by

- CT
- PET-CT
- Any enlarged LN → Biopsy
- Bone Marrow Biopsy

Ann Arbor Staging system used (Discussed previously)

TREATMENT :

- Chemo therapy is Mainstay of treatment

  CHOP-R = Cyclophosphamide + Vincristine + doxorubicin + prednisolone + Rituximab
- Surgery has only secondary role
- Surgical role :
  a) Symptomatic recurrence
  b) Limited gastric disease
  c) Complications

COMPLICATION :

- Bleeding
- Obstruction
- There is 5% chance of perforation
  - If stage IE/IIE – Surgery & remove all gross disease
  - If stage IIIE/IV-Surgery & closure of perforation with tissue for diagnosis

TREATMENT of Gastric MALToma :

1) Early stage with no t(11:18) or BCL-10 expression → H. Pylori Eradication with careful follow-up for regression
   - ➢ Repeat Endoscopy @ 2 months to ensure clearance

- ➢ Biannual surveillance for 3 years to look for tumor regression

2) ➢ Transmural invasion
- ➢ Nodal disease
- ➢ Large cell phenotype transformation
- ➢ t(11:18)
- ➢ BCL-10 expression
- ➢ H. Pylori negative

} Predict failure after H. Pylori eradication alone Suggest poor prognosis

Treatment in these cases : Chemo-Radiation +/- Surgery

Small Intestinal Lymphoma

- M/C intestinal neoplasia in children < 10 years.
- M/C in ileum where greatest concentration of gut associated lymphoid tissue (GALT) is present (GALT constitute 80% of Body's lymphatics).
- Perforation more common than in stomach, less bleeding.

TREATMENT :

- In Absence of symptoms - chemotherapy.
- B-cell lymphomas more chemo sensitive than T cell.
- T cell lymphoma : Surgical resection, as more likely to perforate.
- So also in symptomatic cases → Surgical resection.

✡✡✡

Chapter 7 Gastro-intestinal Stromal Tumour (GIST)

- M/C sarcomatous/mesenchymal tumour of GI tract.
- Arises from Interstitial cell → of Cajal the Pacemaker cell.
- May occur anywhere in GIT.
- M/C location : Stomach > SI > LI.
- Vary in pathology from benign to malignant.
- Pathology : It consists of : Smooth muscle cells + neuro-endocrine cells, it also contains spindle cells & epithelioid cells.
- Immune-histo-chemistry (IHC) markers → CD-117 (C kit), CD-34, Actin & myosin & DOG-1.

Gastric GIST

- 50 years, M>F
- Majority arise de-novo
- Rarely as a part of familial Syndrome :
  - ➢ Carneys triad in familial GIST-Paraganglionoma Syndrome (additionally chondroma)
  - ➢ Von-Hipel Lindau Syndrome
  - ➢ NeuroFibromatosis-1 (NF-1)

SIGNS/SYMPTOMS :

May be asymptomatic

Majority symptomatic :

- M/C : GI bleed & pain.
- Bleeding : Malena > Hematemesis.
- Rupture with Intra abdominal haemorrhage → Surgical emergency.

DIAGNOSIS :

- OGDscopy & biopsy
- EUS
- CECT

STAGING :

AJCC TNM Staging system used

T1 : < 2 cm

T2 : > 2, < 5 cm

T3 : > 5 cm, < 10 cm

T4 : > 10 cm

N1 : nodal metastasis present

M1: distal metastasis present

Mitotic Index (MI) : Low < 5/50 hpf, high > 5/50 hpf

Estimation of malignant potential :

Size	MI	Risk
< 5 cm	< 5/50 hpf	Low
5-10 cm	< 5/50 hpf	Intermediate
> 10 cm	> 5/50 hpf	high

TREATMENT :

Surgery is mainstay of treatment, options include :

- Wide Local excision
- Sleeve gastrectomy
- Partial/total gastrectomy
- En-block resection in advanced cases
- Margin of 1 cm required.

- LN metastasis unusual, **therefore regional lymphadenectomy not recommended.**
- Recurrence is common, it could be either metastatic (M/C in liver) or local or both.
- Therefore follow up is warranted.
- Adjuvant chemotherapy → Imatinib Mesylate (glevac)

  Its a tyrosine kinase KIT inhibitor

  Sunitinib is used in imatinib resistant cases

Resectable tumour

↓

Resect

↓ Low Risk (< 3 cm MI < 5) → Surveillance

↓ Moderate to high risk to recurrence (> 3 cm MI > 5) → Adjuvant imatinib

---

Unresectable tumour

↓

Neo Adjuvant Imatinib

↓

Restaging

↓ Resectable → Surgery & Adjuvant imatinib (1 year)

↓ Unresectable → imatinib 400 mg daily – Indefinately

Small Intestinal GIST :

- M/C in jejunum & ileum.
- 50-60 year, M>F.
- Malignant GIST are > 5 cm at diagnosis in 50%.
- Arise from muscularis propria & usually grow extra murally with spread to Adjacent organs.
- Commonly cause :
  - Obstruction
  - Bleeding

  } requiring urgent surgery
- Metastasis : Hematogenously to liver, lung, bone
- LN metastasis : Unusual
- Prognostic Indicators : Size, mitotic index.

Estimation of malignant potential :

Size	MI	Risk
< 2 cm	< 5/50 hpf	Low
2-5 cm	< 5/50 hpf	Intermediate
> 5 cm	> 5/50 hpf	high

TREATMENT :

- Segmental resection.
- Lymphadenectomy not necessary.
- followed by Adjuvant Imatinib.
- Imatinib could also be given as neo adjuvant therapy followed by surgical resection in advanced cases.

✡✡✡

NOTES

SECTION II

Hepato-Pancreatico-Biliary Oncology

Chapter 8

Hepatocellular Carcinoma

- M/C Primary malignancy of liver.
- M/C Solid organ cancer
- M/C Cause of death in patient with cirrhosis

ETIOLOGY :

1) Virus:

   HBV
   - Integrate into DNA → cause mutation
   - Chronic inflammation → cirrhosis → Ca

   HCV
   - RNA virus → do not integrate into DNA
   - Chronic inflammation → cirrhosis → Ca

   Risk of Ca due to HBV increases if :

   a) Patient is a carrier

   b) Vertically transmitted infection (*i.e.* perinatal)

   c) Acquired in childhood

2) Alcohol abuse → cirrhosis → Ca
3) Smoking
4) Aflatoxin – Produced by fungus (Aspergillus) when it grows over grains and peanuts.
5) Thorotrast – Thorium dioxide containing dye previously used for angiography

   It also increases risk of :

   a) hepatic fibrosis

b) Angiosarcoma

c) Cholangio carcinoma

6) Anabolic Steroids, OC pills

7) Autoimmune hepatitis

8) NAFLD : non alcoholic fatty liver disease

9) Metabolic disorders : a) Haemochromatosis

b) Wilson's disease

c) α-1 antitrypsin deficiency

SIGNS/SYMPTOMS :

1) Right upper quadrant pain.

2) Anorexia, nausea, vomiting.

3) Per abdominal examination may reveal a lump in right hypochondrium.

4) If intraperitoneal rupture occurs : Severe pain + shock

5) If it compresses Bile duct : Obstructive jaundice

6) If it Involves vessels →
- Portal vein thrombosis
- Hepatic vein thrombosis (Budd chiari syndrome)

7) Hemobilia

8) If associated with cirrhosis → features of decompensation

9) Paraneoplastic syndrome :
- Hypercholesterolemia (M/C)
- Hypercalcemia
- Hypoglycemia
- Erythrocytosis

INVESTIGATION :

a) USG (Abdomen + Pelvis) :

- For screening in high risk patients
- Can diagnose early stage HCC

b) CECT (Abdomen + Pelvis)/MRI :

- Helps in definitive diagnosis and treatment planning.
- **Significant features of malignancy on CT :** ***Enhancing in arterial phase with early wash out of contrast in venous phase.***
- *Other features to be noted:*

1) Hypervascularity
2) Extent of disease – on basis of arterial phase images
3) Peritoneal metastasis
4) Nodal metastasis
5) Vascular involvement
6) Thrombus in portal/Hepatic venous system
7) Biliary involvement

c) PET scan :

- To rule out extrahepatic disease (if indeterminate on CT/MRI and if resection is to be planned)
- For identifying Bone mets for which it is better than bone scan

d) Tumour markers :

Alfa feto protein (AFP) levels :

- > 20 ng/ml – Sensitive to predict HCC (False positive in chronic active viral hepatitis)

  > 400 ng/ml – Specific for HCC

- It is used as an adjunctive test for liver mass
- Used for monitoring treated patients for recurrence.
- Lectin fraction 3 of AFP (AFP-L3) is highly specific for HCC

Others : PIVKA, glycipan-3, HepPar-1

Guidelines for diagnosis :

a) EASL – Barcelona - European Association for study of liver.

b) AASLD – American association for study of liver disease

c) Pathological diagnosis – International Working Party criteria

EASL guidelines for diagnosis :

a) Hepatic nodule in USG :

< 1 cm	: repeat USG at 4 months
stable size	: repeat USG at 4 months
increasing size	: manage as per size

b) Hepatic nodule 1-2 cm

↓

Triple phase CT and MRI scan

→ Typical features on one or both **(Enhancing in arterial phase with early wash out of contrast in delayed phase)** ↓ Diagnosis confirmed

→ atypical features ↓ Biopsy for confirming diagnosis

c) ***Hepatic nodule*** > 2 cm

↓

USG – typical features, AFP > 200 ng/ml

↓

CT or MRI

↓ Typical features → ↓ Diagnosis confirmed

↓ atypical features → ↓ Biopsy for confirming diagnosis

d) ***For patient with high risk for HCC***

If lesion found on imaging with/without increase in AFP : consider diagnosis as HCC and start Treatment

e) ***For patient with low risk***

Biopsy to confirm diagnosis

Risks associated with percutaneous FNA of liver tumour :

a) Tumour spillage
b) Rupture/bleeding in subcapsular tumour/cirrhosis

HCC largely metastasizes to Lung, Bone, Peritoneum :

a) Related history should be asked.
b) X ray chest essential – as lung mets may be present without symptoms.
c) Bone scan – only if symptoms are present.
d) For peritoneal mets & locally advanced disease : assessment with Staging laproscopy.

Staging of liver tumour :

STAGING includes : a) Extent of disease
b) Extent of cirrhosis

1) TNM Staging :

- Not used as it does not predict survival.
- It relies on pathology.
- It does not consider liver function tests.

2) Okuda Staging :

Adds up single point for :

a) Tumour **M**orphology : involving > 50% of liver
b) Presence of **A**scites
c) **A**lbumin level < 3 g/dl
d) **B**ilirubin level > 3 mg/dl

This staging system distinguishes patient with poor prognosis from patient with potential long term survival.

(Pneumonic MAAB)

3) CLIP : (Cancer of Liver Italian Program)

a. **P**ortal vein thrombosis	No Yes		0 1
b. **A**FP (ng/dl)	< 400 > 400		0 1
c. **C**hild pugh class	A B C		0 1 2

d. Tumour morphology	Uni Multi Massive	< 50% < 50% > 50%	0 1 2

Score – 0-3 : Potential for survival

Score – 4-6 : Advanced disease

(Pneumonic : PACT)

4) CUPI – Chinese University Prognostic Index

Applies mainly for HBV related HCC.

5) Barcelona Clinic Liver Cancer System (BCLC) :

	No. of tumour	Size	Liver function	Performance status	Other features/ signs of PHT	Threatment option
Very early stage	1	< 3 cm	good	good	No	• Ideal candidate for LT • Excellent prognosis • 75% survival
Early stage **BCLC A**	< 3 or Single	each < 3 cm	good	good	No	• LR • LT • Percutaneous ablation • 50-75% survival
Intermediate Stage **BCLC B**	> 3	each > 3 cm	good	good	No EHD No vascular invasion	Palliative therapy Chemo-embolization
Advanced Stage **BCLC C**			good		• Mild Ca related symptom (+) • EHD (+) • Vascular Invasion (+)	• Prognosis Poor • Sorafenib

	No. of tumour	Size	Liver function	Performance status	Other features/ signs of PHT	Treatment option
Terminal Stage BCLC D	Poor Great tumour burden				Severe cancer related symptom	Symptom Palliation

LR = liver resection LT = liver transplant EHD = extra-hepatic disease PHT = portal hypertension

Factors to be assessed before deciding Treatment :

- ***Patient factors :***
  a) Performance status (ECOG grade)
     0 – Fully active
     1 – Ambulatory, able to carry light weight, sedentary work
     2 – Ambulatory with all self care possible
     3 – Limited self care
     4 – Completely disabled
     5 – Moribund
  b) Constitutional symptoms (fatigue, wt loss)

- ***Assessment of tumour :***
  a) Extent of tumour : Number and size of lesion
  b) Serum AFP
  c) Vascular invasion
  d) Extrahepatic disease
  e) H/o previous tumour rupture and bleeding

- ***Assessment of underlying liver disease :***
  a) Presence or Absence of underlying disease
  b) Severity of underlying disease
     ➪ Child pugh grade : A/B/C

- PHT : Present/absent
  Severity of PHT

c) Volume of remnant liver

d) Architecture of remnant liver

e) Functional assessment of remnant liver is essential part of work-up CT & MRI helps in this assessment

PATHOLOGY :

- Histologically : It may be well/moderate/poorly differentiated. This however does not predict outcome

Gross:

a) Hanging type:
   - Connected to liver by small vascular stalk, easily resectable without loss of adjacent non-neoplastic liver tissue

b) Pushing type:
   - Well demarcated, contains a fibrous capsule
   - Growth displaces vascular structures
   - Majority resectable

c) Infiltrative type:
   - Infiltrate surrounding structure even if of small size

d) Multifocal
   - Starts as single tumour,
   - Multiple satellite lesions secondary to portal vein invasion and metastasis.

TREATMENT :

Liver resection or liver transplant are the only available curative treatment options

Therapeutic Option:

1) **Surgery :**

- Liver Resection → Open
  → Lap
- Liver Transplant → Cadaveric
  → Live

(All of the above) Chance of Cure 50-75% 5 year survival

2) **Trans arterial therapy** –
   - Embolization (TAE)
   - Chemoembolization (TACE)
   - Radio embolization (TARE)

3) **Percutaneous therapy:**

- Chemical ablation :
  - ➢ Ethanol
  - ➢ Acetic acid
- Thermal ablation :
  - ➢ Radio frequency (RFA)
  - ➢ Laser
  - ➢ Microwave
  - ➢ Cryoablation
- Nonthermal - Non-chemical
  - ➢ Irreversible electroporation
  - ➢ Light activated drug therapy
  - ➢ High intensity focus ultrasound (HIFU)

4) **Systemic therapy :** • Sorafenib

- Chemotherapy
- Radiotherapy

Liver Resection – Done if :
→ No Cirrhosis/Child A cirrhosis
→ No vascular invasion
→ No extra hepatic disease

- Can be done : Open or Laproscopically
- Lap only if : Solitary lesion, < 5 cm
  Located in peripheral segment of liver

↓

Disadvantage :

- High recurrence rates
- Post-op mortality
- Post-op morbidity

Advantage : Better survival rate compared to other modalities.

Liver transplant :

- It's an optimal treatment option as it treats the underlying liver disease along with the HCC.
- Recommended for tumour within **MILAN criteria** with underlying CLD with Portal HTN.
- Resection to be done as per **MILAN criteria:**
  a) 1 lesion < 5 cm
  b) 3 lesion < 3 cm each
  c) No extrahepatic disease
  d) No vascular invasion.

- ***Contraindication :*** a) Extrahepatic spread

  b) Vascular involvement

  c) AFP $\geq$ 10,000

  d) Tumour rupture

<u>Trans arterial therapy</u> :

Mainly used for : Unresectable HCC

BCLC B patients

a) Embolisation with gelfoam — TAE

b) Chemembolization — TACE

- ➢ Based on principle that liver is divided into eight segments with each segment receiving its own blood supply and blood supply to HCC is predominantly Arterial So by cannulating the specific arterial vessels supplying the tumour we can occlude it causing necrosis of tumour tissue without causing systemic toxicity.
- ➢ TACE involves using chemotherapeutic drugs with or without lipoidal.
- \- Lipoidal is an ester derived from poppy seed. Lipoidal is concentrated within the hepatocytes, thus increasing its duration of contact with cancerous hepatocytes.
- ➢ Drugs used : Doxorubicin, Cisplatin, Mitomycin.
- ➢ M/C drug used is: Doxorubicin — DEBDOX-TACE.

  Have good response with low complication rate.
- ➢ **TACE** – Should not be used in patients with :

  a) Poor liver function

  b) Complete portal vein thrombosis

- ***Side effects :***
  - Pain
  - Fever
  - Liver abscess
  - Biliary tract necrosis
  - Acute cholecystitis
  - Gastro-duodenal ulceration
  - Ileus
  - Pancreatitis
  - To prevent side effects use : drug eluding Beads
- Beads used may be either :
  - Polyvinyl microsphere
  - Super absorbent polymer microsphere

c) Embolisation with Radioactive agent (Yttrium-90) (TARE)

- Radioactive microspheres are injected into the tumour feeding artery.
- Can be used for all tumour irrespective of :
  - Site
  - Size
  - Number
- Can also be given in presence of cirrhosis and portal vein thrombosis.
- Can downstage tumour to fall within MILANS criteria *i.e.* as a downstaging/bridging procedure before transplant.
- Can be done as day care procedure.

Percutaneous Ablation technique :

Radiofrequency Ablation :

- Most commonly used ablative technique.
- Electrode inserted into tumour tissue

  ↓

  Alternating electric field generated around it

  ↓

  Due to high tissue electric resistance intense heat generated at tip

  ↓

  This heat energy causes tissue coagulation and death
- Can be done as day care procedure.
- These electrodes can be introduced either
  a) Percutaneously under image guidance
  b) By doing Lap/open surgery
  c) After Resectional Surgery
- It should be used for tumour within milan's criteria, but not suitable for Resection or transplant.
- Good effect for tumour < 3 cm.
- Higher recurrence rate with higher tumour size.
- Ablating with a margin of > 3 mm of surrounding normal tissue decreases recurrence rate.
- It is inferior to Resectional surgery but superior to ethanol injection ablation.
- Can't be used for tumours near surface, near stomach, bowel, Biliary tract, major vessels due to **Heat Sink effect.**

Side effects :

- Tract seeding
- Visceral injury
- A. V. fistula
- Bilioma
- Pneumothorax
- Cholecystitis
- Pseudoaneurysm of hepatic artery
- Liver abscess

<u>Microwave Ablation</u> :

- It involves use of electromagnetic waves of frequency > 900 Hz
- When it passes through the tissue it generates continuous rotation of individual molecules that generates heat resulting in tissue damage.
- Depth and shape of ablation depends upon :
  - Power
  - Frequency
  - Type of needle
- Higher local recurrence compared to RFA
- Superior to RFA in terms that it can be used in tumours with unfavourable location.

<u>Laser Ablation</u> :

- Light energy used to destroy tissue.

Via a fibre-optic wire – Laser introduced in tumour

↓

Light energy generated

↓

Is absorbed by tissue

↓

Tissue destruction

- Area of tissue destroyed depends upon: Power & frequency of laser & duration for which the laser is used
- M/C used light source – Nd : YAG
- Still under trial for small tumours.

Percutaneous ethanol injection :

- Oldest technique
- Ethanol injected into tumour

↓

Induces cell dehydration, denaturation of proteins and occlusion of small vessels.

↓

Tumour tissue necrosis

- Different approaches for administration

low dose multiple session 2-10 ml/session	single session high dose ↓GA	high dose multiple session > 10 ml/session

- Used for tumours in Milan's criteria
  - *Disadvantage :-* rate of recurrence due to inadequate tumour necrosis due to inhomogeneous distribution of ethanol
  - Unlike RFA it can be used for tumours @ unfavourable sites.
- When used simultaneously with other modalities, it might have synergistic effect.

Irreversible Electroporation :

- It is a non thermal ablation technique.

↓

Via electrodes placed into or near target tissue

↓

Short intense electric pulses are delivered that generates electric field in tumour tissues

↓

This electric field alters tumour cell membrane potential

↓

At a critical point cell membrane ruptures

↓

Forming nano pores which allow conduction of electric current

↓

By changing amplitude and duration of current we can reseal this membrane : reversible electroporation

However if very high voltage is applied

↓

It keeps these nanosize pores permanently open

↓

Thus disrupting cell membrane integrity

↓

Cell death

- It causes cell death in micromili seconds.
- Does not affect-tissue scaffolds so can be used for tumours closed to bile duct and blood vessels.
- Generates sharp demarcation zone between ablated and non-ablated tissue, therefore can be monitored in real time by CT/USG.
- To be done under GA and muscle blockade.

  Contraindications :

  - ➢ Pacemaker
  - ➢ Arrhythmia
  - ➢ H/o Ml
  - ➢ H/o epilepsy

Light Activated Drug Therapy :

- Aptocine (Talaporfine Na) – a light sensitive, water soluble, semi synthetic drug molecule derived from a chlorophyll derivate.
- Under Image guidance, a flexible wire containing LED at its tip is inserted into tumour and Aptocine is injected intravenously.

Aptocine is specifically concentrated by tumour cell.

↓

Activation of Aptocine by light

↓

Generation of free O_2 radicals

↓

Causes Apoptosis

- ↓ Immune Response
- ↓ Vascular Occlusion
- ↓ Cell death

- Activated Aptocine destroys cells irrespective of cell cycle.
- CD8 cells generated even attack cells that share antigen with tumour tissue.
- No risk of photosensitivity.
- No serious side effect.

HIFU :

- High intensity Ultrasound waves are used.
- They focus waves from a distant site onto a focal point.

  Where it generates heat that causes coagulation necrosis of tissue.
- The waves pass through intact intervening tissue.
- It needs to be focussed accurately.
- ***Advantage:***
  - ➢ No radiation
  - ➢ No Surgery
  - ➢ No need to introduce electrodes therefore not invasive

  - So can be used multiple times.

- ***Disadvantage:***
  - Difficult to use while patient is breathing so patient to be ventilated for controlled breathing.
  - Can't be used for lesions near rib as bone reflects the ultrasound waves.

Sorafenib :

- For BCLC stage C

  i.e. Advanced stage tumour with good liver function *i.e.* child-A cirrhotic.
- Acts via Ras signalling pathway.
- ***Side effects*** –
  - Hand foot syndrome
  - Hypertension
  - Skin rash
  - Enteritis
  - Fatigue

Chemotherapy :

- Only Doxorubicin has shown benefit in advanced HCC.
- No hormonal agent proven to be of benefit yet.

Radiotherapy :

- Insufficient – evidence for internal/external beam Radiotherapy use.
- Used only for cases not suitable for any other form of treatment.

- Radiotherapy itself causes Radiation induced liver disease (RILD).
- **RILD** – anicteric hepatomegaly + Ascites + increased liver enzymes within 2 weeks following irradiation.
- In Severe cases : liver failure.

- Newer modalities :
  - 3D conformal Radiotherapy
  - Intensity modulated Radiotherapy
  - Stereotactic body Radiotherapy
  - Proton therapy

  } decreases radiation induced hepato-toxicity

  - SHORT: Stereotactic Hypofractionated Radiotherapy.

Fabro lamellar HCC

- Occurs in young adults without cirrhosis.
- M=F
- Not encapsulated but well circumscribed & slow growing, therefore high resectability with better prognosis.
- Pathology : central fibrotic scar, causing confusion with FNH.
- Calcification and heterogeneous enhancement on CT helps differentiate.
- AFP not elevated.
- Tumour marker : Neurotensin.
- High resectability with better prognosis.
- However recurrence is common after surgery.

✡✡✡

Chapter 9

Adenocarcinoma of Pancreas

- Ca with dismal prognosis with 5 year survival <5%
- M > F, highest incidence in 6th decade

ETIOLOGY :

1) Smoking : There is a linear association between cancer risk and smoking pack years with risk persisting for many years after smoking cessation
2) Chronic pancreatitis
3) Diabetes
4) Occupational
5) Obesity
6) Prior cholecystectomy

} Controversial

7) Hereditary :
   - Hereditary Pancreatitis : due to PRSS1 mutation
   - FAP : APC gene mutation.
   - HNPCC → Mismatch Repair genes mutation.
   - BRCA-2 mutation.
   - Hereditary atypical mole & multiple melanoma syndrome : CDKN-2A gene mutation.
   - Cystic fibrosis.
   - Peutz Jeghers syndrome.

Cancer Progression : (Fig. 9.1)

Tumour progression is from Pan 1A (Columnar metaplasia → Pan 3 (CIS)

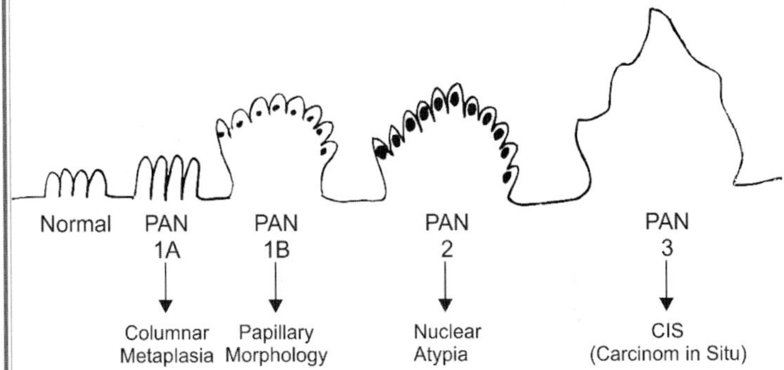

Fig. 9.1: Cancer Progression

Pan 1A → Columnar metaplasia
(Columnar mucinous epithelium without Atypia)
↓
Pan 1B → Papillary architecture
↓
Pan 2 → Increasing nuclear Atypia
↓
Pan 3 → Carcinom in Situ (CIS) with marked cytological Atypia

Cancer Genetics :

- Initiating event most probably is KRAS oncogene activation.
- Tumor suppressor genes like: CDKN-2A, P16, P53. DPC4 → all play a critical role.

PATHOLOGY :

- M/C type is pancreatic ductal adenocarcinoma.
- Usually scirrhous with abundant desmoplastic reaction in

which neoplastic glands are widely scattered.

SIGNS/SYMPTOMS :

- Defining presenting symptom for pancreatic head Ca → Painless progressive jaundice.
- If pain is present it usually is in epigastrium radiating to back
- Others : Weight loss, Anorexia, weakness.
- Ca Body/tail :
    - Usually present in advanced stage with pain & weight loss
    - Present late as there is no specific manifestation
- On examination : Palpable Gall bladder → **Courvoisier's Law**

In Advanced disease :

- Virchows left supra-clavicular lymph nodes
- Sister Joseph umbilical Nodule
- Irish axillary lymph nodes
- Blumers shelf deposits
- Hepatomegaly, Jaundice, Ascites

DIAGNOSIS :

1. **Blood invesigaion :**
    - ➢ Raised Bilirubin and alkaline phosphatase levels resulting from CBD obstruction.
    - ➢ Albumin levels need to be checked pre-op as a part of nutritional assessment.
    - ➢ Tumour markers : CEA, **CA 19-9**, AFP.

      ↓

      Most sensitive & specific marker

- Lack of rise in CA19-9 levels in some patients is due to negative Lewis Antigen status.

2. ***Triple phase contrast enhanced CT***
   - → Non contrast phase
   - → Arterial phase
   - → Portal venous phase

- Provides information for loco regional staging
- Relation to vascular structure
- Metastasis

3. **EUS :**
   - Identifies smaller lesion missed on CECT.
   - Provides information for loco regional staging especially relationship to vascular structures.
   - Advantage → FNAC possible.

4. **ERCP, MRCP, PTC :** Characteristic for periampullary tumours is DOUBLE DUCT SIGN

5. **FDG-PET-CT** → useful to differentiate benign from malignant tumors and identify metastasis

6. **Staging Laproscopy :**

   Decreases the chance of non therapeutic laparotomy.

   Particularly used for Patients with :
   - Tumour > 3 cm
   - Highly elevated Ca 19-9
   - Features of advanced disease such as weight & loss pain

STAGING :

Following biopsy confirmation via EUS-FNA tumour is accurately staged as per AJCC – TNM staging system.

T1 : Intra pancreatic < 2 cm in size

T2 : Intra pancreatic > 2 cm

T3 : Tumour extending beyond pancreas except into Celiac axis, Superior mesentcric artery (SMA)

T4 : Involves Celiac axis, SMA

N1 : Nodal involvement

M1: Metastasis

Staging :

I T1/T2

II T3/N1

III T4

IV M1

→ **Accordingly as per NCCN guidelines tumour can be :**

Resectable :

1) T1, T2, T3 *i.e.* within or just into peri-pancreatic tissue.
2) Without celiac Axis or SMA involvement.
3) With no evidence of Portal vein-SMV Axis involvement.
4) With no evidence of metastasis.

Borderline Resectable :

1) SMV – Portal vein abutment (<180° of vein is in contact with tumour).
2) SMV – Portal vein Encasement (>180° of vein is in contact with tumour).

3) SMV – Portal vein reconstructible short segment occlusion.
4) SMA < 180º Abutment.
5) Reconstructible Abutment/Encasement/occlusion of Hepatic A or GDA.
6) No SMA, celiac Artery involvement.

Un-Resectable :

1) T4 *i.e.* involving SMA, celiac Artery.
2) Stage IV tumour.

TREATMENT :

Surgical resection is the only potentially curative treatment.

For head Ca :

Whipples pancreatico - duodenectomy :

- First performed by Whipples & Parson as a 2 stage procedure.
- First single stage surgery was done by Trimble.
- Pylorus preserving pancreatico (PPPD) was first performed by Longmire-Traverso.

Technique for PPPD* (Fig. 9.2) *:

- Laparotomy.
- Explore to see all peritoneal surfaces for evidence of metastatic disease that would deem it inoperable.
- Extended Kocherisation: done upto left lateral margin of Aorta.
- Infra pancreatic SMV dissected.
- Right Gastro-epiploic vessels & middle colic V. sacrificed
- Cholecystectomy done.

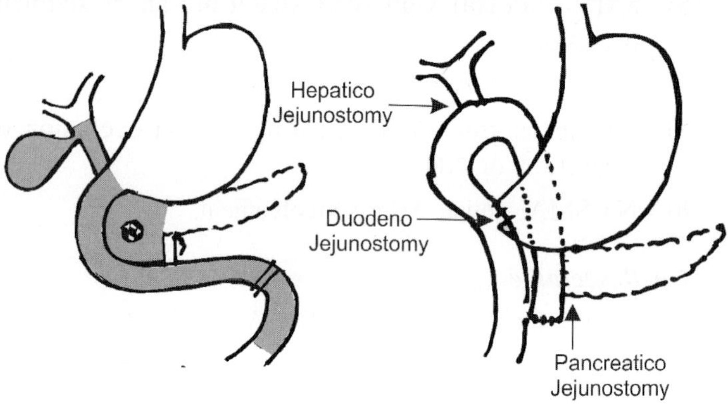

9.2a 9.2b

Fig. 9.2: Technique of PPPD

- HDL dissected, CHD divided.
- GDA blocked & blood flow in HA confirmed.
- Right gastric A & GDA divided.
- Duodenum first part divided 2 cm distal to Pylorus.
- Jejunum divided 10 cm distal to Ligament of treitz.
- Pancreas dissected of SMV - PV.
- 4 point ligation of superior & inferior pancreatico-duodenal artery.
- Pancreas divided at neck.
- Uncinate dissection completed and specimen extracted
- Frozen section.
- Pancreatico jejunostomy (PJ).
- Hepatico jejunostomy (HJ).
- Duodeno jejunostomy (DJ).
- Drains & feeding jejunostomy

- Pancreatico jejunostomy → 2 layer duct to mucosa
- Hepatico jejunostomy → 5-8 cm downstream, single layer, duct to mucosa
- Most important margin : retroperitoneal or uncinate margin

Body & tail :

- These tumours are usually advanced & rarely resectable with short survival
- Treatment → distal pancreatectomy & En-bloc splenectomy
- Contraindication to surgery → involvement of celiac Axis

Controversies :

1) **Pylorus preserving pancreatico duodenectomy (PPPD) vs conventional PD.**

PPPD found to be better than classical PD as per a few studies :

- Is now considered the operation of choice.
- Meant to reduce Bile Reflux & dumping syndrome.

2) ***Pancreatico-jejunostomy:*** **Duct to mucosa vs Dunking.**

In cases where duct cannot be identified, gland can be invaginated into jejunum (Dunking).

3) ***P-J vs P-G (pancreatico-gastrostomy) :*** Still controversial

4) ***Extent of lymphadenectomy***

- Radical lymphadenectomy has been proposed to reduce recurrence (Japan)
- Standard Lymphadenectomy includes : Peripancreatic, Pyloric, and Portal LN
- Radical Lymphadenectomy : In addition it includes

Hilar LN dissection & retroperitoneal dissection from celiac axis above to IMA below, between the two renal hilum.

*5) **Open vs Laproscopic approach:*** Laparoscopy is complex, not widely used

*6) **Antecolic vs Retrocolic D-J :*** Antecolic D-J is said to improve gastric emptying & is commonly done.

Complication of surgery :

Mortality now days are rare.

Morbidity is common & includes :

1) Delayed gastric emptying - M/C complication.
   - Causes decreased tolerance to oral intake requiring prolonged NG decompression.
2) P-J Leak :-
   - Defined as drain output of any measurable volume on or after post-op day three, with amylase value > 3 times the serum value.
   - P-J remains the Achilis heel.
   - Predictive factor : Texture and duct size – leak more with Soft & fatty pancreas with duct size < 3 mm. Leak less with firm pancreas with wide duct.
   - Usually managed by creating a controlled fistula by retaining the intraoperatively placed drain.
   - Rarely additional Drain placement or Surgery with completion pancreatectomy required.
3) Leak from D-J/G-J, H-J : Rare
4) Intra Abdominal Abscess

5) Wound infection
6) Pancreatic insufficiency → Exocrine / Endocrine
7) Re-Exploration
8) Pulmonary-Cardiac complication

- Median survival → 22 months
- Relapse → Local (uncommon) / Metastatic

Adjuvant Chemo Radiation :

Current recommendation:

- Gemcitabine + 5-FU + Radiation
- However usefulness of radiation is being questioned.

Neo-Adj Chemotherapy :

- being used increasingly common.

Rationale :

- It ensures that all patient receive multi – modality therapy.
- Efficacy of chemo is maximised as it is delivered to an intact gland with an established blood supply.
- Response to chemo can be assessed.
- Progression on NACT suggests it to be an aggressive tumor thus we can prevent these patient from undergoing extensive surgery which may not provide any survival benefit.
- Chemotherapy, itself is a physiological stress & helps identify patients who are unlikely to tolerate the stress of surgery.

- It is not possible to give post-op Chemo in up to 25% due to sugical complication or inability to recover physiologically.
- It improves negative margin & LN metastasis status.
- Role is particularly clear in BORDERLINE RESECTABLE tumours.

PALLIATION :

80% have advanced Ca.

Principle : - Non-op therapy to optimise quality of life

Biliary obstruction: - ERCP & stenting with SEMS (self expansile metallic stent) made of Nitinol
- Surgery (Hepatico-jejunostomy) is cheap but less preferred

GOO (Gastric outlet Obstruction) : - Stenting
- Surgery : Lap/open Gastro-jejunostomy

Pain Relief : - Opioid analgesia
- Celiac ganglion block with 0.25% bupivacaine (3 ml) + 10 ml Alcohol

SURVIVAL :

Stage I/II : 15-20 months

Stage III : 6-10 months

Stage IV : 3-6 months

✡✡✡

Chapter 10

Cystic Neoplasm of Pancreas

INTRADUCTAL PAPILLARY MUCINOUS NEOPLASM (IPMN) :

- Also known as mucin-secreting carcinoma, villous adenoma of the duct of Wirsung.
- Seen in 6th to 7th decade, M = F.
- More common in head and uncinate process of the pancreas.

TYPES OF IPMN :

- *Branch duct IPMN :* Involves dilation of the pancreatic duct side branches.
- *Main duct IPMN :* Abnormal cystic dilation of the main pancreatic duct.
- *Mixed-type IPMN :* Side branch IPMN that has extended to involve the main pancreatic duct.

PATHOLOGY :

- Arising within the pancreatic ducts.
- Ductal epithelium forms a papillary projection into the duct.
- Mucin production causes intraluminal cystic dilation of the pancreatic ducts.
- Careful histologic examination of the entire specimen required.

SIGNS/SYMPTOMS :

- Present with abdominal pain or recurrent pancreatitis caused by obstruction of the pancreatic duct by thick mucin

- Some have steatorrhea, diabetes, and weight loss secondary to pancreatic insufficiency.
- Predictors of malignancy (SENDAI consensus guidelines)
  - Main pancreatic duct diameter ≥ 1 cm
  - Cyst size ≥ 3 cm
  - Abnormal cytology
  - Mural nodules
  - Jaundice, diabetes, raised ALP

DIAGNOSIS :

1. Endoscopy :

- Mucus extruding through a large, fish-mouth like papillary orifice is virtually diagnostic.
- **EUS** helps in better characterization of the lesion and allows aspiration of cyst fluid.

2. **CECT:** Dilated main pancreatic duct, cysts of varying sizes, and possibly mural nodules may be seen.
3. **Aspirated fluid analysis :** Mucin-rich aspirate, high CEA and amylase level.

LOCALISATION :

Pre-operative localization is problematic in IPMN because :

- Over production of mucous can cause ductal dilation both proximal and distal to the tumor.
- Tumour tends to spread microscopically along the duct.

TREATMENT :

- Surgical resection is recommended for main duct IPMN, symptomatic and large (>3 cm) branch duct IPMN, or IPMNs with an invasive component

- Observation : For asymptomatic small (< 3 cm) branch duct IPMNs without associated nodularity.

PROGNOSIS :

- Local anatomic resection is essentially curative for branch duct IPMN.
- Recurrence in the remnant gland is seen in upto 10% in main duct IPMN.
- IPMN with invasive carcinoma : 5 and 10-year survival is 60% and 50% (better than pancreatic adenocarcinoma).

MUCINOUS CYSTIC NEOPLASM (MCN):

- M/C cystic neoplasm of the pancreas which can be malignant.
- Usually affects young women.
- M/C in body and tail of pancreas.

PATHOLOGY :

- Grossly are macrocystic.
- MCNs contain mucin-producing epithelium with presence of mucin-rich cells within ovarian-like stroma.
- Estrogen and progesterone receptor staining is positive in most cases.

SIGNS/SYMPTOMS :

- Majority cases now a days are being incidentally diagnosed.
- Vague abdominal pain may be seen in half.
- A subset of patients may have pancreatitis in which case the pancreatic cystic lesion may be misdiagnosed for pseudocyst.

DIAGNOSIS :

- **CT scan :**
  - Characteristic Findings : Solitary cyst with fine septations and rim of calcification.
  - It may not be able to distinguish between benign and malignant MCNs.
- **EUS** helps in better characterization of the lesion and allows aspiration of cyst fluid.
- **Cyst fluid analyses :** Mucin-rich aspirate, high CEA and low amylase levels.

  Fluid analyses can provide accurate diagnosis in up to 80% of cases.

Features suggestive of malignancy :

- Presence of eggshell calcification on cross sectional imaging.
- Larger tumour size.
- Presence of mural nodule.

TREATMENT :

- Exclusion of malignancy is possible by biopsy alone, therefore surgical excision is indicated for all cases.
- Surgical resection is standard treatment for MCN.
- In absence of malignancy, resection is curative and no further surveillance is required.

SEROUS CYSTIC NEOPLASM (SCN) :

- M/C in the head of pancreas.
- Almost exclusively in women.
- Majority benign and have no malignant potential.

PATHOLOGY :

- Grossly SCNs are large & well-circumscribed.
- Are microcystic consisting of small cysts filled with clear fluid.
- Spongelike/Honeycomb appearance.
- Microscopic examination reveals multiloculated, glycogen-rich small cysts.

SIGNS/SYMPTOMS :

- Majority asymptomatic.
- Some may present with vague abdominal pain.
- Lesscommonly : Weight loss and obstructive jaundice.

DIAGNOSIS :

- EUS & CECT.
- Aspiration from cyst yields non-viscous fluid with low CEA and low amylase levels & mucin absent.
- Central calcification gives rise to a characteristic central sunburst, radial, or stellate scar pattern on CT scan.

TREATMENT :

SCN is benign therefore resection is indicated only when diagnosis is in doubt or when they become symptomatic or size > 4 cm.

✡✡✡

Chapter 11

Pancreatic Neuro-Endocrine Tumours (PNET)

INSULINOMA :

- It is insulin producing tumor of pancreas causing "Whipples triad"
  - Hypoglycaemic symptoms on fasting or exercising
  - Low blood sugar levels (< 2.8 mmol/L)
  - Relief on IV glucose
- Most common functioning PNET
- F > M
- Age group : > 50 years
- Evenly distributed in head, body and tail
- Majority solitary, 10% multiple
- Usually benign, < 2 cm, without signs of invasion,
- 10% malignant

ETIOLOGY : Unknown, some cases are associated with MEN-1 syndrome.

SIGNS/SYMPTOMS :

Fasting hypoglycaemia with :

- Neuroglycopenic symptoms : blurred vision, confusion, abnormal behaviour, amnesia, tremors, loss of consciousness & Death.
- Cardiovascular : because of catecholamine release : palpitations, sweating & anxiety.

DIAGNOSIS :

- Gold standard for diagnosis : **72 hours fasting test** : an insulin to glucose ratio of > 0.4 is consistent with insulinoma

  (Raised serum C-peptide levels helps differentiate insulinoma from exogenous factitious hypoglycemia)

LOCALISATION :

Pre-op :

- EUS better than CT/MRI better than USG
- CT/MRI : hyperattenuating because of rich blood supply
- Angiography : characteristic vascular blush seen
- Porta venous sampling for insulin with or without arterial stimulation with calcium

Intra-op :

Exploration and palpation & IOUS (intra-op ultrasound).

DIFERENTIALS :

- Hepatic insufficiency
- Enzymatic deficiency
- Medication/drugs
- Nesidioblastoma in children : hyperplastic islet cells

TREATMENT :

Surgical excision recommended.

Once presence confirmed and relation to duct identified :

- In benign cases : ENUCLEATE.
- If superficial can be done laproscopically.

- For distal tumors, one can consider distal pancreatectomy
- In those in whom tumour could not be localised : Blind resection avoided.
- For malignant disease: Aggressive resection with peripancreatic lymphadenectomy.

Medical management :

1) Diazoxide : - decreases insulin production
2) Chemotherapy : - Streptozocin
   - 5 FU + Doxorubicin

GASTRINOMA (ZES) :

- Zollinger Ellisons Syndrome, consists of :
  1) Fulminant peptic ulcer disease
  2) Recurs inspite of adequate treatment
  3) Resulting from excessive gastrin production from a non beta cell islet tumour
- Second most common functional PNET
- M > F
- Age group : > 50 years
- More than half (60-80%) malignant
- M/C site of metastasis : Liver
- Majority Solitary
- Majority are found in PASSARO'S/Gastrinoma triangle formed by joining the three points including : **(Fig. 11.1)**
  1) Cystic duct and CBD junction
  2) D2-D3 junction
  3) Pancreatic neck-body junction

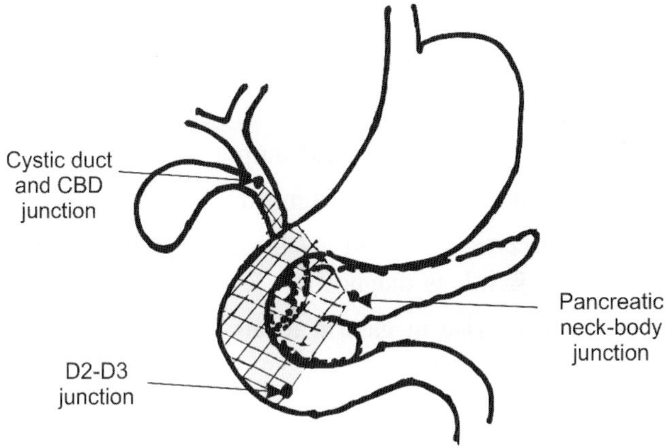

Fig. 11.1: PASSARO'S/Gastrinoma triangle

- Most common site : 1st or 2nd part of duodenum.
- Most common location in pancreas : head of pancreas.
- Pancreatic tumors have worse prognosis compared to duodenal ones.
- There is no way to predict clinical behavior.
- Progression is slow.
- All gastrinomas produce Chromogranin A.

ETIOLOGY :

- Unknown, some cases are associated with MEN1 syndrome.

SIGNS/SYMPTOMS :

- Fulminant peptic ulcer disease.
- With ulcers seen at unusual sites such as esophagus, jejunum.
- Diarrhoea, unique feature of this diarrhoea is that it halts with nasogastric aspiration.

- Abdominal pain.
- GERD.

DIAGNOSIS :

- Gastric pH < 2.5, Basal Acid output (BAO) > 15 meq/hr.
- pH < 2 with high gastrin diagnostic.
- Hypergastrinemia : Gastrin level > 100 pg/mL is suggestive & > 1000 pg/mL is diagnostic.
- Secretin test : rise in gastrin levels by > 200 pg/mL with secretin administration.

DIFERENTIALS :

- Idiopathic PUD/GERD
- Idiopathic chronic Diarrhoea
- GOO
- Atrophic gastritis
- Gastric resection

LOCALISATION :

Pre-op localisation :

- Pancreatic ones are usually > 1 cm in size compared to duodenal tumours which are usually smaller in size.
- Therefore duodenal tumors are difficult to localize compared to pancreatic ones.
- Modalities :
  - Somatostatin Receptor Scintigraphy : Imaging test of choice
  - Others : EUS > CT/MRI/USG.

Intra-op localisation : IOUS.

TREATMENT :

Surgical resection is advised

- Most pancreatic gastrinoma are solitary & in head → Enucleation with pancreatic LN dissection if possible, or else pancreatico-duodenectomy
- Body/tail tumors
  - Enucleation
  - Distal pancreatectomy
- Check duodenum

Duodenal tumours :

duodenum opened longitudinally & wall palpated.

- < 5 mm tumour : enucleated with overlying mucosa.
- > 5 mm tumour : full thickness excision.

Medical management :

1) Octeotide decreases Acid secretion.
2) Proton Pump Inhibitor (PPI) : pantoprazole.

Chemotherapy : Streptozocin
(+) Doxorubicin
(+) 5 FU

Nonfunctional PET :

- No clinical syndrome until disease has advanced.
- IHC markers → positive for chromogranin A, Synaptophysin.
- Usually large : > 5 cm
- Sporadic cases are usually : unifocal
- MEN1 cases are usually : multifocal.

- Usually in head
- Majority malignant
- Compared to functional ones prognosis is worse because of :
  - Late diagnosis
  - Larger size
  - higher malignancy risk
- Tumour marker :
  - Chromogranin A
  - Pancreatic Polypeptide

Deterentia Diagnosis : Adeno Ca.

LOCALISATION :

- EUS, IOUS, CT, MRI.
- Somatostatin Receptor Scintigraphy : newer modality.

TREATMENT :

- Surgical resection, even in presence of distant mets.
- Target at a 'R0' resection.

Glucagonoma :

- Hyperglycemic Cutaneous Syndrome.
- F>M, majority solitary, large, malignant, located in body and tail of pancreas.
- Classic presentation of the 4Ds : Diabetes, dermatitis, DVT, and depression.
- Dermatitis : Necrolytic erythema migrans (M/C manifestation of the disease).
- Diagnosis : Fasting glucagon level > 50 pmol/L.
- Easily localized by CT.

- SRS performed if CT is not informative.
- Treatment : Resection is the treatment of choice.
- Dacarbazine is uniquely effective against glucagonoma.

VIPomas :

- Verner-Morrison Syndrome, Pancreatic cholera.
- WDHA syndrome (watery diarrhea, hypokalemia, achlorhydria).
- Majority solitary, large, malignant, located in tail of pancreas.
- Constant features are diarrhea, hypovolemia, hypokalemia and acidosis.
- Variable features are achlorhydria or hypochlorhydria, hyperglycemia and flushing.
- Easily localized by CT.
- **Treatment :** Aggressive preoperative hydration and correction of electrolyte abnormalities and acid-base disturbances. Octreotide is commonly used pre operatively to reduce diarrhea volume.
- Resection is the treatment of choice.

Somatostatinoma :

- M=F, 50 years, majority solitary, large, malignant, located in head of pancreas
- Causes steatorrhea, mild diabetes, cholelithiasis and hypochlorhydria
- Easily localized by CT
- Treatment : Resection is the treatment of choice

- In unresectable disease, octreotide and interferon alfa may improve symptoms.

NOTE :

All pancreatic cancers and neoplastic cysts are most common in pancreatic head except :

- MCN and Glucagonoma : M/C in body and tail
- VIPoma : M/C in Tail
- Insulinoma : Equally distributed in head, body and tail

✡✡✡

Chapter 12

Carcinoma Gall Bladder

- Aggressive & with poor prognosis with majority having an advanced disease.
- 60-70 years,
- F > M,
- Common in northern India, Pakistan.
- Earliest genetic mutation: p53 loss of function

ETIOLOGY :

Theory for etiology : Chronic inflammation progressing to cellular proliferation

1) Gallstones → risk higher with stones > 3 cm
   Type of stone → no correlation
2) Choledochal cyst
3) PSC (Primary sclerosing Cholangitis)
4) APBJ (Anomalous pancreatico-biliary junction)

} chronic inflammation

Others :

1) GB polyps : risk higher with polyp > 1 cm.
2) Porcelain GB.

PATHOLOGY :

- Adenocarcinoma : most common.
- Progresses from dysplasia → CIS → invasive Ca.
- Most are systemic with nodal disease & distant metastasis at diagnosis.
- Morphological subtypes:
  - Infiltrative

- Nodular
- Papillary

- Papillary subtype are usually
  - Indolent & limited to GB and hence have good prognosis
- Infiltrative subtype has worst prognosis

SPREAD :

1) Nodal spread → first to cystic LN → pericholedochal and periportal LN → retro and peripancreatic LN → aorto-caval LN
2) Hepatic spread: because of venous drainage spread directly to seg IV.
3) Trans peritoneal carcinomatosis or notoriously along biopsy or surgical wound tracts..

SIGNS/SYMPTOMS :

- Symptoms usually occur in advanced stage, they include :

  Right hypochondriac pain, chronic epigastric pain, weight loss, jaundice, mass, early satiety.
- It may present with Acute Cholecystitis due to neck obstruction

  Presents early. better prognosis.
- Chronic cholecystitis.

DIAGNOSIS :

1) **USG :** 1st Investigation for any patient with right hypochondriac pain.

   Finding :
   - ➢ Heterogeneous mass in GB lumen
   - ➢ Asymmetrically thickened GB wall
   - ➢ Polyp > 10 mm should raise suspicion

2) CT :

- Tri-phasic CECT done.
- Loco regional Staging.
- Identifies vascular involvement, LN & peritoneal metastasis.
- Sensitivity for detection of liver infiltration is however poor.

3) Cholangiography :

ERCP, MRCP, PTC } In Obstructive Jaundice

4) EUS

- Provides information for loco regional staging
- Advantage → FNAC possible.

5) PET scan:

- Role emerging
- Helps identify extrahepatic spread, thus avoiding a fruitless surgery

6) Tissue diagnosis :

Percutaneous transhepatic biopsy or EUS guided FNA may be obtained in unresectable cases such as Portal vein encasement or extensive hepatic involvement or metastasis.

7) Tumour marker : CA19-9

8) Others:

Serologic biomarkers can potentially differentiate between cholelithiasis and Ca: CA242 and CA125

STAGING :

AJCC – TNM staging system is used

T1a : Limited to lamina propria (there is no sub-mucosa)

T1b : Limited to muscularis

T2 : Limited to perimuscular connective tissue without infiltrating serosa/liver

T3 : Perforating serosa, penetrating liver OR one extra hepatic organ

T4 : Into main PV, HA OR $\geq$ 2 extrahepatic tissue

N1 : Peri-portal, peri-ductal LN involvement

N2 : Celiac, para-Aortic, para-caval LN involvement

M1 : Metastasis present

Stages :

I T1

II T2

III T3/N1

IV T4/N2/M1

Other staging systems : Nevin's classification

TREATMENT :

- Surgery is only potential for cure.
- There are 4 specific patient subgroups.

1) GB polyp :

- Therapy is cholecystotomy by open method.
- Accidental puncture during a lap cholecystectomy may convert a potentially curable Ca into an incurable one.

2) GB Ca detected after cholecystectomy :

Depends on T stage :

a) **T1a** → Lamina propria → only cholecystectomy sufficient.

b) **T1b** → Muscularis : cholecystectomy sufficient as long as R0 resection achieved.

   - In case of vascular, Lymphatic involvement or PNI (peri neural invasion) :
     Extended Cholecystectomy aiming at R0.

c) **T2** → Radical cholecystectomy

- ***Extended Cholecystectomy*** includes : **(Fig. 12.1)**
  - Wedge hepatic resection with 2 cm margin.
  - Cystic duct stump clearance which may require resection of extra hepatic Bile duct.
  - Lymphadenectomy :
    - Cystic duct LN

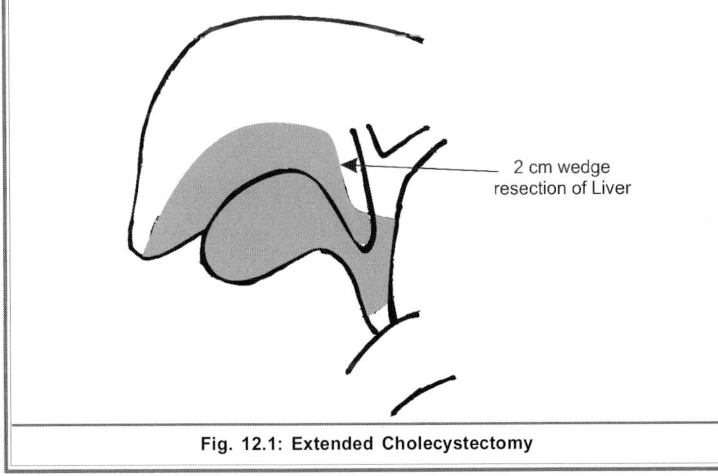

Fig. 12.1: Extended Cholecystectomy

- Peri-choledochal & Peri-portal LN
- Pancreatico-duodenal LN

- Port site excision : is controversial

- ***Radical Cholecystectomy*** includes :
  - Resection of liver segments IV b and V
  - At times may require a central hepatectomy (seg IV, V & VIII) or rarely a right trisectionectomy
  - Resection of extra hepatic bile duct.
  - Enbloc Resection of all invaded tissue to achieve R_0.
  - Radical Lymphadenectomy.

3) **Pre-op diagnosis of Ca GB** :
   - Offered Surgery if no e/o metastasis.
   - Because only surgery can offer cure.
   - Begin with a diagnostic laproscopy (staging).
   - Metastasis would preclude surgery & would direct the treatment towards non-op palliation.
   - Debulking has no role.
   - Majority are **T3 & T4** tumour → Radical cholecystectomy

4) **Advanced disease** → Palliation

Principle for palliation	:	Non-op treatment to optimise quality of life
Biliary obstruction (associated with poor prognosis)	:	ERCP & stenting with SEMS (self expansile metallic stent) made of Nitinol Surgery (hepatico-jejunostomy) is cheap but less preferred
GOO (Gastric outlet Obstruction)	:	Stenting Surgery (gastro-jejunostomy)
Pain Relief	:	Opioid analgesia Celiac ganglion block with 0.25% bupivacaine (3 ml) + 10 ml Alcohol
Chemotherapy	:	Gemcitabine + Cisplatin

✡✡✡

Chapter 13

Cholangio-Carcinoma

- Tumours arising from bile duct epithelium
- Rare with dismal prognosis
- Proximal : Intrahepatic or peri-hilar, account for 2/3rd cases
  Hilar cholangio Ca also known as Klatskin tumour is M/C type
- Middle : Rare
- Distal : Periampulary

Bismuth corlette classification used for Klatskin tumour **(Fig. 13.1)**

Type I : Limited to the common hepatic duct, below the level of the confluence

Type II : Involves the confluence of the right and left hepatic ducts

Type IIIa : Type II and extending into right hepatic duct

Type IIIb : Type II and extending into left hepatic duct

Type IV : Tumour Hilar extending into both hepatic duct

ETIOLOGY :

Theory for etiology : Chronic inflammation progressing to cellular proliferation.

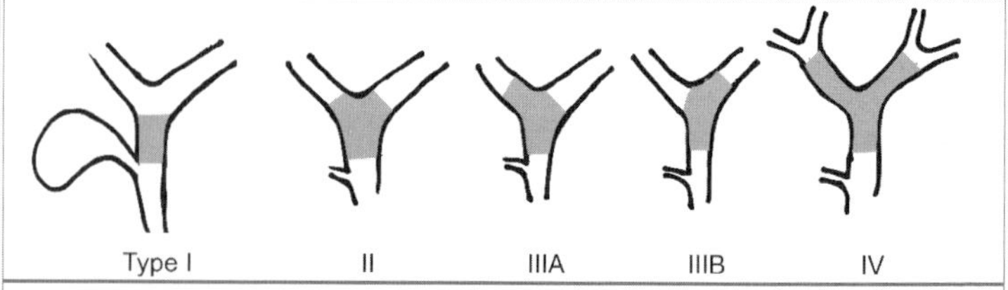

Fig. 13.1: Bismuth corlette

1) Choledochal cyst: Due to exposure to toxic pancreatic secretions.
2) APBJ: Anomalous pancreatico-biliary junction.
3) PSC: Primary sclerosing Cholangitis : Autoimmune etiology with, Multiple ductal strictures.
4) Liver flukes: Clonorchis sinesis & Opisthorvhis Viverni → Inflammation with ductul strictures & obstruction
5) RPC: Recurrent Pyogenic Cholangitis → Recurrent CBD stones & ductal strictures
6) Choledocholithiasis: Bile duct stones
7) OCPs
8) Thorotrast
9) Smoking

} Chemical carcinogens (items 7–9)

PATHOLOGY :

3 Pathological subtypes :

1) Sclerosing type :
   - Usually this type is seen in proximal duct
   - Concentric periductal fibrosis with circumferential duct occlusion
   - Full extent of tumour misjudged because of periductal inflammation
   - No defined mass formation
2) Nodular type → Firm mass growing into lumen
   - Usually in distal CBD
3) Papillary type → usually in distal CBD
   - Polypoidal soft growth, slowly progressive with better prognosis

90% Cholangiocarcinoma are Adenocarcinoma - usually mucin producing

Precursor lesions :

a) Biliary intra-epithelial neoplasia

b) Intra-ductal papillary neoplasia

SIGNS/SYMPTOMS :

If at bile duct confluence or below:

- Pain less jaundice due to obstruction at or below bile duct bifurcation
- High coloured urine
- Pruritus
- Clay coloured stools
- Steatorrhea, fat soluble vitamin deficiency (A, D, E, K).
- Present earlier with better prognosis.

If above confluence :

- Unilobar obstruction → unilobar atrophy with contralateral hypertrophy → delayed presentation.

DIAGNOSIS :

1) Blood investigstions

- Increased bilirubin, Alkaline phosphatase
- Coagulation profile
Albumin } Deranged if Long standing
- Tumour markers : CEA, CA 19-9 : unreliable for diagnosis, better for surveillance.

2) USG :

- Hilar Cholangio Ca: IHBRD with decompressed EHBD
- Peri-ampulary CholangioCa : IHBRD with dilated EHBD

  (IHBRD = intra hepatic bile radical dilatation)

  (EHBD = extra hepatic bile duct)

3) Triple phase CT :

- Locoregional staging & identification of vascular involvement.
- Helps in pre-op planning.

4) Cholangiography :

- ERCP, MRCP, PTC main role is to define proximal extent of tumour.
- ERCP however carries risk of cholangitis.
- Establishment of tissue diagnosis is not necessary for surgery.
- Indicated in cases of unresectable tumor

STAGING :

TNM staging of Klatskin tumour :

T1 : Limited within the wall of CBD

T2a : Invading Peri-CBD connective tissue

T2b : Invading liver parenchyma.

T3 : Unilateral hepatic artery & portal vein involvement

T4 : Main branch hepatic artery & portal vein involvement
Bilateral secondary biliary radical involvement

N1 : Peri-ductal, Peri-portal LN involvement

N2 : Coeliac, para-aortic, para-caval LN involvement

M1 : Metastasis present

PROGNOSIS :

Prognosis better with T1, T2, N0 disease with R0 resection.

TREATMENT :

- Complete R0 resection with reestablishment of biliary-enteric drainage is the only treatment modality that can result in long-term patient survival.
- As of now transplantation has no role
- **Contraindications to Surgery:**
  - Involvement of the main portal vein
  - Bilateral (B/L) involvement of either hepatic arterial or portal venous branches
  - B/L spread up to secondary biliary radicles
  - Unilateral (U/L) hepatic artery involvement with extensive contralateral (C/L) ductal spread
  - U/L lobar atrophy with C/L portal venous or secondary biliary radicle involvement
  - N2/M1 disease.
- Staging laparoscopy may be used to prevent nontherapeutic laparotomy.
- Operative strategy changes depending on tumor location within the biliary tree.

1. **Distal CholangioCa:** Whipples Pancreatico-duodenectomy.

2. **Middle third CholangioCa**: Radical Choledochectomy which includes bile duct resection with regional lymphadenectomy.

3. **Proximal CholangioCa :**
   - En-bloc resection of extra-hepatic bile duct (EHBD) with hepatic Resection & regional lymphadenectomy to achieve R0.
   - The addition of major hepatectomy that includes segment IV and the caudate lobe has led to improved R0 rates.

Treatment For Klatskin Tumour as per Bismuth Corlette class:

Type I:

- Radical Choledochectomy with atleast 1 cm margin
- Margins to be checked by frozen section

Type II & IIIa:

- Right Trisectionectomy including caudate lobectomy

Type IIIb:

- Left Hepatectomy including caudate lobectomy

Type IV: are usually non-resectable.

- Vascular resection of PV & HA followed by reconstruction is now feasible surgical option for locally advanced tumour
- Large volume liver resection with low FLR (future liver remnant) can lead to PHLF (post hepatectomy liver failure)

- **Measures to increase FLR volume**:
  - Portal vein embolization (PVE)
  - Associating liver partition and portal vein ligaton for staged hepatectomy (ALPPS)
  - Target FLR: >20% in normal liver, >30% in fatty liver, >40% in cirrhotic liver

- **Parenchyma preserving hepatectomy**:
  - Parenchyma adjacent to the hepatic hilum including segment I, IVb, V resected,
  - Data emerging.

- **Pre-op Biliary Decompression (PBD)**
  - Role of PBD and best way to achieve it is controversial with data still emerging.
  - In setting of complete biliary obstruction, hepatic resection carries additional risk of bleeding and sepsis.
  - Stenting of future liver remnant in such cases has found to improve prognosis
  - Percutaneous trans-hepatic biliary drainage (PTBD) and endoscopic Naso-biliary drainage (NBD) are preferred over ERCP and stenting
  - Indications:
    1) Bilirubin level > 10 mg/dL
    2) Prolonged time expected between presentation & resection
  - Target bilirubin level 3 mg/dL

- **Adjuvant Chemo Rx:**
  - For patients with nodal disease, or R1 resection.

- Gemcitabine + Cisplatin
- Same regimen used for palliation in advanced disease

- **Palliation:**
  - Obstructive jaundice: ERCP & stenting / PTBD
  - SEMS used if life expectancy > 6 months
  - Pain: Narcotics, Celiac plexus block
  - Duodenal obstruction: Stenting

✡✡✡

NOTES

SECTION III

GENITO-URINARY ONCOLOGY

Chapter 14 Renal Cell Carcinoma

- RCC/Adenocarcinoma of kidney.
- M:F 2:1
- M/C in 5th – 6th decade of life.
- Black men – higher incidence.
- Asians – Lower incidence.

ETIOLOGY :

- **Sporadic :**
  - ➢ Cigarette smoking.
  - ➢ Occpational exposure to asbestos, solvents, cadmium.

- **Hereditary :**
  - ➢ Von Hippel Lindau syndrome (VHL)
    - Cerebellar hemangioblastoma
    - Retinal angiomata
    - Bilateral clear cell RCC
  - ➢ Hereditary papillary RCC
  - ➢ Birt Hugg Dube syndrome.
- Acquired cystic disease of kidney.
- Long term renal insufficiency requiring hemodialysis. M/C with peritoneal dialysis

Cancer Genetics : Structural changes in chromosome 3p noted.

PATHOLOGY :

- It arises from proximal tubular epithelium, arises in cortex with equal frequency in upper and lower poles.

- It arises from cortex, so grows out into the perinephric tissue causing characteristic bulge and mass effect.

Gross :

- Yellow to Orange (due to abundant lipids).
- Do not have a true capsule but have pseudocapsule consisting of compressed renal parenchyma, fibrous tissue with inflammatory cells.
- Tumour usually has areas of necrosis, cystic degeneration & hemorrhage

Pathological types :

1. Conventional clear cell type – Rounded/polygonal cells with abundant cytoplasm rich in :
   - Cholesterol
   - Triglycerides
   - Glycogen
2. Papillary (chromophilic) –
   - Less glycogen and lipids
   - Cytoplasm contains mainly mitochondria and cytosome.
   - Granular cytoplasm
3. Oncocytic type – Packed with mitochondria, have a granular appearance.
4. Chromophobe type – Reticulated cytoplasm.
5. Collecting duct type – Irregular border, basophilic cytoplasm, extensive anaplasia, invade blood vessel with infarction of tissue.

6. Neuroendocrine type.
7. Unclassified.

M/C type :

Mixed with clear cell, granular cell & sarcomatoid appearing cells.

SPREAD :

- RCC is a highly vascular tumour, spreads by :-
  - Direct invasion through renal capsule into perinephric and adjacent structures.
  - Direct invasion into renal vein.
- M/C site of distant metastasis – Lung.
- In Bones – it causes osteolytic metastases.

SIGNS/SYMPTOMS :

- Hematuria (painless) M/C
- Sometimes clot colic
- Flank pain
- Flank mass
- Cough } suggesting
- Bone pain } metastatic disease
- Paraneoplastic syndrome :
  - Erythrocytosis : Renal hypoxia resulting in increased erythropoietin production.
    (30% have normochromic anemia)
  - Hypertension, refractory to antihypertensive, resulting from increasing rennin levels.

- ➢ Hypercalcemia (Parathormone related peptide-PTH-r-P).
- ➢ **Stauffer syndrome**. Non-metastatic hepatic dysfunction.
  - Due to overproduction of GM – CSF by tumour.
  - Raised liver enzymes & bilirubin, deranged PT – INR, hypoalbuminemia.
- ➢ Fever, fatigue, weight loss.

DIAGNOSIS :

- **USG –**
  - ➢ First investigation done for hematuria.
  - ➢ Differentiates solid from cystic lesions.
- **CECT –**
  - ➢ Lesion appears hypodense with heterogenous pattern of enhancement with IV contrast.
  - ➢ Most sensitive test for renal mases.
- **MRI** – Primary advantage is in detecting IVC involvement
- **CT angiography/MR angiography –**
  - ➢ to identify arterial anatomy.
  - ➢ to see extent of vascular involvement.

  Conventional angiography – not routinely done.
- **Radionuclide study** – Bone scan for assessing metastasis.
- **FDG – PET**
  - ➢ For assessing response to systemic therapy in metastatic disease.
  - ➢ For progression/recurrence.

Benign solid renal lesion may be mistaken for RCC.

Features suggestive of malignant & not benign disease :

- Size > 7 cm
- No interface between tumour and renal parenchyma.
- Amputation of collecting duct.
- Involvement of perinephric fat and adjacent structures.
- Lymphadenopathy and distant metastases.
- Calcification.

STAGING :

TNM staging system used (compare to Adrenal Ca staging).

T1 – Tumour less than 7 cm, within kidney

T1a – < 4 cm

T1b – 4-7 cm

T2 – Tumour > 7 cm limited to kidney

T3 –
- Invades perinephric tissue, adrenals within gerota's fascia (T3a)
- Renal vein, IVC (below diaphragm) (T3b)
- IVC above diaphragm (T3c)

T4 – Invades beyond gerota's fascia

N1 – Single node involved

N2 – More than 1 node involved

M0 – Distant metastasis absent

M1 – Present

- Original staging system used previously was – Robson staging – no prognostic value.
- Fuhrman grading used for renal tumour grading –

- 4 grades based on nuclear size, irregularity, nudeolar prominence.

TREATMENT :

- Surgical excision is the only curative therapeutic option in localised disease
- Appropriate staging required prior to planning surgery
- **Radical nephrectomy :** For T1, T2, T3a, T3b
  - It involves :
    1. Enbloc removal of kidney and its Gerota's fascia.
    2. Ipsilateral adrenal gland
    3. Half of ureter
    4. Lymph nodes upto area of transection of renal vessels.
  - **Incision :**
    1. Unilateral chevron
    2. Thoraco abdominal
    3. Typical flank incision
    4. Mid line incision.
  - **Laparoscopic approach** may be attempted in localised renal tumour (< 10 cm in size without local extension or renal vein/caval thrombus).
- **For caval thrombus :**
  - Tumour thrombus usually does not invade caval wall – therefore easily removable.
  - Treatment depends on cephalad extension.
  - For T3b – Tumour involving renal vein/IVC below hepatic vein – radical nephrectomy with thrombectomy should suffice.

- If it extends upto right atrium (T3c) – Cardiopulmonary bypass required prior to attempt at removal.

- **Partial nephrectomy:**
  - For tumours < 4 cm in size
  - Involves wedge resection of tumour with adequate margin of normal renal parenchyma.
  - Approach: - Open
    - Laparoscopic
    - Bench surgery f/b autotransplantation

- **In case of Bilateral RCC or Solitary kidney lesion**

↓

Radical nephrectomy

↓

Long term dialysis or Renal transplant

- Alternative ⟶ Partial nephrectomy

- If multiple lesions present *e.g.* : VHL disease
  - Enucleation.
  - Cryoablation with liquid N_2/Argon – percutaneously – under MRI guidance.
  - Radio frequency ablation (RFA).
- Very large tumour – Renal artery embolization – Angio infarction → down-sizing
  - It is also palliative for patients with non-Resectable tumour with symptoms.
- If locally recurrs – repeat resection
- Old age with comorbidities – Cryoablation, RFA
- Old patient with tumour < 3 cm – Observation.

- Disseminated disease :

  Nephrectomy – open or laparoscopy recommended for cytoredution, to : - Relieve pain
  - Control severe hemorrhage

- Renal carcinoma with :
  - Surgically resectable solitary lung metastasis
  - Surgically resectable solitary bone metastasis

  } Nephrectomy + Resect the solitary metastases

- Radiation therapy –
  - Used as neo adjuvant/adjuvant therapy.
  - RCC is relatively radioresistant
  - Can be used as palliative measure for metastatic disease.

- Biologic response modifiers :
  - Recombinant Interferon alpha (IFN α)
    - Subcutaneous injection 3-5 days/week.
    - Most likely beneficial after tumour burden removed with only nodal and distant metastases remaining.
  - Recombinant IL – 2 – Approved by US FDA for Advanced renal carcinoma.

- **Newer biologic agents :**
  - Sorafenib and Sunitinib:- Approved for advanced RCC.
  - Others : Bevacizumab, Temsirolimus

- **Rationale for use**

Sporadic/inherited tumour → Deletion of VHL gene

↓

Activation of hypoxia inducible factor (HIF)

↓

Sorafenib → { Increased VEGF ← Bevacizumab; Decreased PDGF ← Sunitinib; m TOR ← Temsirolimus }

↓

Promotes Angiogenesis

↓

Hypervascular nature of RCC

FOLLOW-UP & PROGNOSIS :

- T1 : Yearly F/U with x-ray chest, LFT, RFT
- T2, T3 : 3 monthly/6 monthly F/U
- If partial nephrectomy – F/U with repeat CECT
- 5 year survival for : T1 – 100%

  T3 – 60%

✡✡✡

Chapter 15

Nephroblastoma/ Wilm's Tumour

- M/C solid tumour of childhood
- No sex predilection
- Peak age :- 3rd year of life
- In 5% of cases tumour is bilateral
- Alteration in WT_1 – chromosome 11p

ETIOLOGY :

Majority : non familial : sporadic

<u>Familial cases</u>: 1% of all cases. They include :

- **WAGR syndrome :**
  - Wilms tumour
  - Aniridia
  - Genitourinary malformation
  - Retardation

- **Beckwith – Wiedemann syndrome :**

  (Overgrowth disorder)

  Features
  - Macroglossia
  - Macrosomia
  - Abdominal wall defect : omphalocele, exomphalos
  - Hemihypertrophy
  - Hypoglycemia

- **Trisomy 18**

- **Denys Drash syndrome :**
  - Gonadal dysgenesis
  - Nephropathy
  - Wilms tumour

GENETICS :

KNUDSONS – 2 hit hypothesis.

- 2 hits (mutation) to DNA required before a tumour could develop
  - Sporadic – 2 postzygotic mutations required for tumour formation
  - Familial – 1 prezygotic mutation and subsequent post zygotic event required for tumour formation. (the first insult is inherited in DNA and second insult occurring post zygotically leading to cancer).
- Therefore sporadic cases occurs at older age.
- Familial occurs at young age and tends to be bilateral.

PATHOLOGY :

- Precursor lesion – Nephrogenic rest (NR)
- Typical Wilms tumour consist of :-
  - → Blastemal elements (aggressive)
  - → Epithelial elements (less aggressive, better prognosis)
  - → Stromal elements
- **Unfavorable features :**
  - Focal/diffuse element of anaplastic cells.
    - Diffuse worse than focal
  - Clear cell, rhabdoid elements.

- **Favorable features :**
  - Blastemal, epithelial, stromal elements without anaplasia.

Gross :

Large, multilobulated, gray/tan coloured with focal areas of hemorrhage and necrosis with fibrous pseudocapsule.

SPREAD :

Distant metastasis more common:

- M/C to lungs (85-95%)
- Liver (10-15%)
- Bones

SIGNS/SYMPTOMS :

- Present with an abdominal lump
- Abdominal distension
- Abdominal pain
- Nausea, vomiting, fever, hematuria.

DIAGNOSIS :

- Clinical examination
- CECT
- MRI
- Needle biopsy - only if tumour is very large with resection not possible in order to give pre-op chemotherapy/ radiotherapy.

D/D :

1. Hydronephrosis
2. Polycystic kidney disease

3. Neuroblastoma.
    - Arising from adrenal gland/paraspinal ganglion
    - Usually cross midline.
    - Causes outward and downward displacement of kidney (drooping lily sign on IVP)
    - High frequency of calcification and metastasis.
    - Tumour marker : VMA, cathecolamine

STAGING :

- National Wilms Tumour Study Group (NWTS) staging system used.
- It is a post operative staging system, *i.e.* staging done after surgical resection.

Stage I:

- Tumour limited to kidney, capsule intact and no invasion of renal sinus.
- No spillage before/after excision.
- Complete excision with no residual tissue.

Stage II :

- Tumour extending beyond kidney, penetrating capsule reaching upto renal sinus.
- Spillage before/after surgery occurs.
- Complete excision possible.

Stage III :

Non-hematogenous tumour residue.

- Lymph node metastases.
- Peritoneal metastases – Tumour spillage beyond flanks
  Peritoneal implants

- Infiltration of surrounding vital structure.
- Gross/microscopic residual tissue left after excision.

Stage IV :

- Hematogenous dissemination to lung, liver and bone.

Stage V :

- Bilateral renal involvement.

TREATMENT :

Multimodality therapy

- → Surgery
- → Chemotherapy
- → Radiotherapy

- Wilm's tumour is both chemo and radiosensitive
- Treatment is based on stage & histology

Surgery :

1. Unilateral Wilms tumour, resectable (not crossing midline/ involving adjacent viscera).

Go for surgical resection.

Principles :

- ➢ No need of retroperitoneal lymphadenectomy.
- ➢ Biopsy of regional lymphatics (renal hilar, para aortic nodes).
- ➢ Careful examination of opposite kidney and rest of abdomen.
- ➢ Intra caval thrombus – remove.
- ➢ If extending to adjacent organs – if possible resect.

- Avoid tumour spillage – leads to recurrence.

2. ***Bilateral wilm's tumour :***

Biopsy for diagnosis and staging
↓
Neo-adjuvant chemotherapy
↓
Renal sparing surgery

Stage-wise Treatment:

Stage	Histology	Treatment
Stage I	favourable/anaplastic	Surgery + chemotherapy (vincristine + dactinomycin) No radiotherapy
Stage II	favourable	
Stage III Stage IV	Favourable →	Surgery + chemo (vincristine + dactinomycin + doxorubiun) + radiotherapy
Stage II Stage III Stage IV	Anaplastic	Surgery + chemo (vincristine + dactinomycin + doxorubiun) + radiotherapy + Cyclophosphamide + etoposide (salvage chemo regimen)

Stage V → biopsy followed by chemo **6-8 weeks** → reassess → renal sparing procedure.

- Post-op Radiotherapy additionally recommended in:
  - Clear cell histology
  - All stage of rhabdoid tumour.

Prognosis : 4 years survival – 90%

Poor outcome – unfavourable histology
- → Anaplastic
- → Clear cell histology
- → Rhabdoid

Chapter 16

Bladder Carcinoma

- Age : > 65 years
- M > F

ETIOLOGY :

1. Cigarette smoking - dose related.

   Cause : α and β naphthylamine secreted in urine of smokers.

2. Occupational exposure – chemical, dye, rubber, petroleum, leather, printing industry.

   Due to exposure to :
   - Benzidine
   - β-naphthylamine
   - 4-aminobiphenyl

3. Cyclophosphamide.
4. Ingestion of artificial sweeteners.
5. Physical trauma to urothelium :
   - Infection
   - Instrumentation
   - Calculi

Genetics :

- Loss of genetic material on chromosome 9- early event in bladder Ca development.

  It's a "field defect" occurring throughout urothelium.

- P_{53} deletion.
- Increasing expression of C-Ha-ras, chromosome 11_p.
- Deletion of 17_p.

PATHOLOGY :

1. **M/C type : Transitional cell carcinoma** (98% cases)

- **Types** : Papillary, Exophytic → Superficial; Sessile, Ulcerated → Invasive

- **Carcinoma in situ (CIS)** – Anaplastic cell layer – with loss of normal cellular polarity.
  - ➢ Cells contain large irregular hyperchromatic nuclei prominent nucleoli.
  - ➢ Grossly : – angry looking, red velvety with dilated veins

2. **Non-transitional cell carcinoma**

   Mixed, undifferentiated, squamous cell carcinoma, adeno-carcinoma

- **Squamous cell carcinoma :**
  - ➢ Associated with history of chronic infection.
  - ➢ Vesical calculi
  - ➢ Chronic catheter use
  - ➢ Associated with Bilharzial infection due to Schistosoma Hematobium
  - ➢ Often nodular and invasive, poorly differentiated.

- **Adenocarcinoma :**
  - ➢ Preceded by cystitis with metaplasia.

   - HPR : mucus secreting cells with glandular/colloid/ signet ring pattern.
   - Primary adenoCa : usually arises in base of bladder.
   - AdenoCa arising from urachus : dome of bladder.

- **Mixed :**
   - Composed of combination of transitional & squamous cell type.
   - Poorly differentiated.

- **Undifferentiated :**
   - No mature epithelium.
   - Neuroendocrine features or small cell carcinoma features.
   - Are aggressive in nature.

The most common tumour metastizing to bladder :

1. Melanoma
2. Lymphoma.

SYMPTOMS :

- Gross/microscopic intermittent hematuria (M/C).
- Diffuse CIS – frequency, urgency, dysuria mimicking UTI
- Advanced disease :
   - Flank pain due to retroperitoneal metastases or ureteral obstruction
   - Bone pain, due to bony mets

SIGNS :

- Large volume tumour – palpable mass on bimanual examination

- If immobile – suggests adherence to adjacent structures.
- Hepatomegaly.
- Supraclavicular lymphadenopathy.
- Lower limb lymphedema due to pelvic lymphadenopathy.
- Metastasis to skin presents with painful nodules with ulceration.

DIAGNOSIS :

a. Lab findings :

1. Urine examination – Hematuria.
2. Urine cytology for exfoliated cells,
   - ➢ Yield improved by irrigating bladder with isotonic saline.
   - ➢ Detection rate high in CIS, high grade/high stage tumour.
3. Azotemia if tumour obstructs ureteric orifice
4. Anaemia –
   - ➢ Chronic blood loss
   - ➢ Bone marrow invasion.
5. Markers for bladder cancer
   - ➢ BTA (bladder tumour antigen)
   - ➢ Methylated markers
   - ➢ NMP 22 (nuclear matrix protein)
   - ➢ Increasing micro RNA
   - ➢ MCM (minichromosone maintenance protein)
   - ➢ **Lewis x antigen on exfoliated cells**
   - ➢ **Telomerase activity in exfoliated cells**

b. Cystoscopy with biopsy :

- CIS – flat area with erythema with irregularity & angry looking dilated veins — Biopsy & cauterize it.
- Superficial tumours appear as multiple papillary lesions
- High grade appear as large sessile tumours

} Cystoscopic Resection

- Fluorescent cystoscopy with blue light – hematoporphyrin instilled into bladder. These derivatives gets accumulated in cancer cells. They are detected as glowing red under fluorescent light.

c. CT
d. MRI

} To examine upper urinary tract.
To identify local extent & help in loco-regional staging
To rule out metastasis.

e. Bone scan if Alkaline phosphatase raised.

STAGING :

TNM staging system used

Ta – confined to lining epithelium – no invasion of BM.

T1 – extending to submucosa

T2 – extending to muscularis → T2a (Superficial); T2b (Deep)

T3 – extending subserosa/perivesical tissue

T4 – extending to adjacent structures

→ 4a contiguous organ invasion *e.g.* Prostate, vagina

→ 4b pelvic/abdominal wall (frozen pelvis).

N1 – < 2 cm, single node involved

N2 – N2a : 2-5 cm, single node involved

N2b : < 5 cm, multiple nodes involved

N3 – > 5 cm, multiple node involved

M0 – Distant metastasis absent

M1 – Present.

TREATMENT :

Stage wise treatment :

1. ***Ta :*** Superficial papillary tumour.

- ***TUR :*** Trans urethral resection.

  → Single, non recurrent Low/moderate grade → TUR followed by surveillance or TUR followed by single dose of intravesical mitomycin – C

  → Multiple, recurrent, large High grade → TUR followed by intravesical chemo/immunotherapy followed by Surveillance

2. ***Tis :*** Intravesical chemo/immunotherapy – if does not respond : Cystectomy – no role of radiotherapy

3. ***T1 :*** - TUR followed by intravesical chemo/immunotherapy or

- TUR followed by repeat scopy after 6 weeks
- Regular surveillance must.
- Recurrence = Radical Cystectomy

- **High grade T1 with concomitant – CIS** = Radical Cystectomy

4. T2, T3, T4 :

- All cases with muscle invasion requires definite therapy.
- Options :
  - Radical cystectomy.
  - Radial cystectomy followed by chemotherapy.

- Neo adjuvant chemotherapy followed by radical Cystectomy or external beam radiotherapy.
- Concomitant chemo-radiation.

5. **Any T, N+, M+** → Systemic chemo f/b selective surgery/ irradiation

Surgery :

A) TUR :

- Initial treatment for all bladder carcinoma.
- Done with resectoscope followed by multiple loop resection from base of tumour (if bladder perforates : surgery & close rent with delayed foley catheter reomoval).
- We can estimate tumour stage/grade.
- Disease status after 3 months is a reliable predictor of recurrence and progression.
- Can be considered as definitive therapy in old age with comorbidities.

B) Partial cystectomy :

Mainly for :

- Adenocarcinoma
- Tumours confined to lateral wall/posterior wall
- T1 – T3 tumours

Preoperatively rule out diffuse CIS/tumours by random bladder biopsy.

C) Radical cystectomy with bilateral pelvic LN dissection followed by urinary diversion :

In males – bladder with perivesical fat and peritoneal

attachments with prostate and seminal vesicle excised.

Females – bladder with perivesical fat with peritoneal attachments with uterus, cervix, anterior vaginal vault, ovary and urethra excised.

Chemotherapy :

- ***Adjuvant chemotherapeutic drugs :***

  MVAC : Methotrexate, vinblastine, doxorubicin, cisplatin.

- ***Neo adjuvant therapy :*** CG – cisplatin, gemcitabine

Intravesical chemotherapy :

- Chemotherapeutic agents directly instilled into bladder via catheter.
- Avoids complications of systemic chemotherapy.
- **Role**

  Along with TUR → Adjunctive → prevent reimplantation

  After complete TUR → Prophylactic → to prevent/delay recurrence or progression.

  After incomplete TUR → Therapeutic → cure residual disease.
- Therapeutic Intravesical chemotherapy : given weekly for 6 weeks.
- Prophylactic Intravesical chemotherapy : single dose following TUR.
- Efficacy increased by increasing drug concentration and contact time :
  - By restricting fluids before administration.
  - Patient positioning during treatment

- Avoid instillation of air.
- Avoid urinating for next 1–2 hours.

• **Agents used :**

- ***Mitomycin – C*** - antitumour alkylating antibiotic agent that inhibits DNA synthesis.

  Side effect : 1) Irritative voiding symptoms.

  2) Rash on palm and genitalia

- ***Thiotepa*** - *alkylating agent*

  Side effect : 1) Cystitis.

  2) Myelo suppression

- ***BCG :***

  - Attenuated strain of Mycobacterium Bovis used.
  - Action is immunologically mediated.
  - Mucosal ulceration and granuloma formation can occur.
  - Most effective against – CIS – most effective agent for CIS

    High grade superficial tumours
  - Prevent recurrence
  - Delays progression
  - Protocol : BCG instillation weekly for 6 weeks.

    followed by no BCG for 6 weeks.
  - Maintenance therapy – 3 instillation weekly for 3 weeks followed by 3–6 months interval for 3 years.

Side effect :

1. Hemorrhagic cystitis :
   - treatment – Isoniazid +/- Rifampicin + Vit-B6
   - Stop instillations or dose of BCG reduced

2. BCG sepsis –

- high fever, chills, confusion, hypotension, respiratory failure, jaundice
- Treatment: HRE (Isoniazid + Rifampicin + Ethambutol) + prednisone.

Radiotherapy :

5000-7000 CGY over a period of 6-8 weeks.

- For advance carcinoma, muscle invasive carcinoma.
- When unfit for surgery due to old age/comorbidities.

✡✡✡

Chapter 17 Testicular Tumours

- Right > left.
- Seen in 4th decade of life.
- M/C Primary tumour of testis : Seminoma.
- M/C testicular tumour in infant and children upto 3 years : Yolk sac tumour
- M/C testicular tumour in pre-pubertal children : Teratoma
- 2% Bilateral.
- M/C B/L tumour of testis - Malignant lymphoma.
- M/C primary B/L tumour - Seminoma.
- Genomic change found in all germ cell tumours : an isochromosome of short arm of chromosome 12.

ETIOLOGY :

- Exact cause unknown.
- Strongest association is with Cryptorchid testis.
- 10% cancers develop in patients with H/o cryptorchidism - M/C seminoma.

Others :

- H/o contralateral testicular tumour.
- Exogenous estrogen administration to mother during pregnancy.
- Trauma.
- Infection related testicular atrophy.
- Klinefelters syndrome.
- Testicular feminising syndrome.

Model of Tumorigenesis :

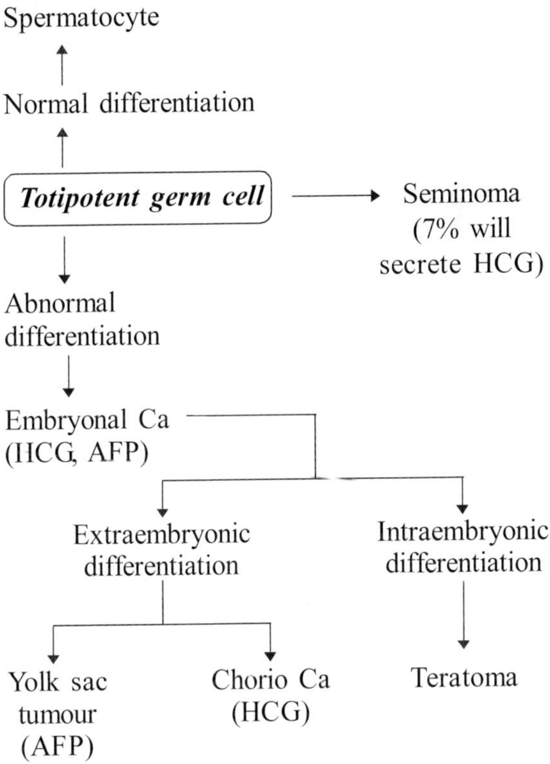

SPREAD :

Germ Cell tumour (GCT) spreads by both lymphatic & hematogenous routes.

- Lymphatic spread is step wise

  1st LN involved in right sided tumours – Inter Aortocaval

  1st LN involved in left sided tumours – Left para aortic

- (Rt) can cross over to (Lt).

  (Lt) can never cross over to (Rt).

Once Tunica albuginea OR Scrotum involved → metastasis to Inguinal LN

Once Epididymis OR Spermatic cord involved → metastasis to external iliac LN, Obturator LN

- Distant metastasis → lung > Liver, Brain.

CLASSIFICATION :

Germ cell tumour (GCT) (90-95%)

- ***Seminoma (35%)***
    - Classical (85%)
    - Anaplastic
    - Spermatocytic

- ***Non-seminomatous Germ Cell Tumour (NGCT)***
    - Embryonal (20%)
    - Teratoma (5%)
    - Choriocarcinoma (1%)
    - Yolk sac tumour
    - Mixed (40%)

Non-Germ cell tumour :

- Leydig cell tumour
- Sertoli cell tumour
- Gonadoblastoma
- Lymphoma

Seminoma :

Age group : 40-50 years.

Pathology :

Gross :

- Cut surface — Homogenous / Pinkish cream colour
- Compresses neighbouring testicular tissue.

Microscopy :

- Oval cells with clear cytoplasm with large round nuclei with prominent acidophilic nucleoli.
- Sheets of cells separated by fine fibrous stroma resembling spermatocyte.
- Contain lymphocytic Infiltrate.

Variants :

- Anaplastic.
- Spermatocytic seminoma – cells resemble different phases of maturing spermatogonia.

Spread :

- hematogenous – uncommon
- Lymphatic metastasis – common

Teratoma :

- Yellow in colour.
- Heterogenous with both solid & cystic components.
- Tumour contains cystic spaces filled with gelatinous fluid

lined by cells which arise from more than 1 germ cell layer, which may be in various stages of maturation and differentiation.

Types :

a) Mature – contain well differentiated tissues arising from ectoderm, endoderm, mesoderm.

b) Immature – contain incompletely differentiated primitive tissue

Embryonal Carcinoma :

a) Infantile type :

- Also known as ***yolk sac tumour/endodermal sinus tumour***.
- M/C in infants and children.
- Characteristic **schiller - duval bodies** seen.

b) Adult type :

- Marked pleomorphism, mitotic figures, giant cells with extensive hemorrhage and necrosis seen.
- **Embryoid bodies** (resembling 1-2 week old embryo with surrounding Syncytiotrophoblast and cytotrophoblasts) seen.

Chorio Carcinoma :

- Consist of cytotrophoblast and syncytiotrophoblast –
- Aggressive in nature
- Early hematogenous spread seen

Interstitial Cell Tumour :

- Well circumscribed, small tumours.
- 10% malignant.

Leydig cell	Sertoli cell
Masculinises	Feminises
Mainly prepubertal	Mainly post pubertal

SYMPTOMS OF TESTICULAR CA:

a) Painless lump, progressively increasing in size (M/C).

Rarely sudden increase in size with severe pain in case of acute haemorrhage into the tumour.

b) Increase in size to 2-3 times normal size – Sensation of heaviness.

c) Loss of testicular sensation.

d) Trauma usually brings it into notice.

Features of Metastasis :

a) Abdominal pain with lump in epigastrium.

b) Cough, dyspnoea, haemoptysis (pulmonary mets).

SIGNS :

- Intratesticular solid mass palpable.
- Epididymis may not be palpable seperately as it may be incorporated in the growth.
- Vas is never thickened.
- Lax secondary hydrocoele may be present in 5-10%.
- PR usually Normal.

- Gynaecomastia in 5% NSGCT.
- Majority of seminoma are confined to testis at time of presentation, whereas majority NSGCT have widespread metastasis at presentation.

DIAGNOSIS :

a) USG – - Mandatory in all suspected cases.
- Opposite testis also to be examined.

b) Blood investigation :

Tumour Markers :

- Used to monitor response to treatment.
- To reassess after orchidectomy, to confirm whether all tumour tissue has been removed.

1. **AFP :** - Increases in Yolk sac tumour, embryonal carcinoma and teratoma (YET).
   - Doesn't increase in pure choriocarcinoma and pure seminoma.
2. **HCG :** Increases in all choriocarcinomas, 50% embryonal carcinoma and 5-10% of pure seminoma (CES).
3. **LDH:** Not a specific tumour marker. Useful as a marker for "bulk'of disease.
4. **PLAP (Placental alkaline phosphatase) :**
   - Useful as a marker for "bulk'of disease.
   - Elevated in seminoma.
5. **GGT (Gamma glutamyl transpeptidase) :**
   Useful as a marker for "bulk'of disease.

c) **FNAC** is Contraindicated as scrotal seedlings may occur resulting in inguinal LN metastasis.

D/D :

1) Epididymitis.
2) Epididymo-orchitis.
3) Hydrocele.
4) Spermatocele.
5) Hematocele.
6) Granulomatous orchitis.
7) Epidermoid cyst : to be differentiated from teratoma.
8) Varicocele.

STAGING :

T

Tis : Intraductal carcinoma (Treatment – External beam radiotherapy)

T1 : Confined to testis and epididymis.
No vascular invasion.

T2 : Involvement of tunica vaginalis/vascular invasion.

T3 : Involvement of Spermatic Cord.

T4 : Involvement of Scrotum.

N

N1 : Involvement of Retroperitoneal lymphnode
< 2 cm, < 6 LNs positive

N2 : Involvement of Retroperitoneal lymphnode
> 2 cm, < 5 cm, > 6 LNs positive

N3 : > 5 cm in size

M

M1a: Pulmonary metastasis, Non-regional LN metastasis.

M1b: Visceral metastasis other than lung.

S

	LDH	HCG mIU/ml	AFP ng/ml
S_1	< 1.5 x (N)	< 5000	< 1000
S_2	1.5-10 x (N)	5,000-50,000	1,000-10,000
S_3	> 10 x (N)	> 50,000	> 10,000

TNMS Staging by AJCC :

IA : T_1

IB : T_2, T_3, T_4

IIA : N_1, S_0/S_1

IIB : N_2, S_0/S_1

IIC : N_3, S_0/S_1

III : M_1 S_2/S_3

Older Staging : — by Bodvin & Gibb

Stage A : Confined to testis

Stage B : Involving regional LN

Stage C : Spread beyond retroperitoneal LNs

TREATMENT :

- First thing to do is : ORCHIDECTOMY
- In suspected testicular tumour : *Chevassu manoeuvre* :
  - Inguinal Incision.

- ➢ Spermatic cord displayed and soft clamp applied.
- ➢ Testis mobilised into wound.
- ➢ Testis bisected along anterior convexity, suspicious area biopsied and sent for frozen section.
- ➢ If malignant, cord double transfixed & divided at level of internal inguinal ring and testis removed.

- After orchidectomy imaging done for staging : X-ray chest, CECT abdomen.
- Repeat AFP, HCG to confirm complete removal of tumour tissue.

Stage wise treatment for seminoma :

IA : T_1 : Radiation therapy

IB : T_2, T_3, T_4: Radiation therapy

IIA : N_1, S_0/S_1 : Radiation therapy

IIB : N_2, S_0/S_1 : Radiation therapy

IIC : N_3, S_0/S_1 : Chemotherapy

III : M_1 S_2/S_3 : Chemotherapy

Is : Only serum tumour markers are raised (S1 to S3) : Chemotherapy

Stage wise treatment for NSGCT :

IA : T_1 : Retroperitoneal Lymph Node Dissection (RPLND) or observation

IB : T_2, T_3, T_4 : RPLND

IIA : N_1, S_0/S_1 : RPLND or chemotherapy followed by RPLND

IIB : N_2, S_0/S_1 : RPLND ± adjuvant chemotherapy or chemotherapy followed by RPLND

IIC : N_3, S_0/S_1 : Chemotherapy followed by RPLND

III : M_1 S_2/S_3 : Chemotherapy +/- resection

Is : Only serum tumour markers are raised (S1 to S3) : Chemotherapy

Chemotherapy : Bleomycin + Etoposide + Cisplatin (BEP)

Testicular Carcinoma in Situ (CIS) Intratubular Germ Cell Neoplasia (ITGCN) :

Preinvasive precursor of all testicular GCTs except :

- *Spermatocytic seminoma*
- *Yolk sac tumor*
- *Teratoma in children*

Progression of ITGCN to invasive disease may take upto 15 years.

ETIOLOGY :

Same as that for GCT.

PATHOLOGY :

- ITGCN cells are located on the basement membrane of the seminiferous tubule and possess morphologic features of malignancy.
- Occasionally the whole tubule may be filled with ITGCN cells.

SIGNS/SYMPTOMS :

Testis is usually normal to palpation.

DIAGNOSIS :

- There is no established tumor marker for CIS, and testicular ultrasound is not reliable.
- Testicular biopsy remains the "gold standard".
- Testis biopsy reliably diagnoses ITGCN because the ITGCN is almost always found throughout the testis.

TREATMENT :

- Treatment options include observation, radiation therapy, and orchidectomy.
- Chemotherapy so far appears to be ineffective against ITGCN.

✡✡✡

Chapter 18

Prostate Cancer

- M/C malignant tumours of men.
- Age > 65 years.
- Prostate Ca in younger men usually associated with positive family history.
- Ca usually arises in peripheral zone **(Fig. 18.1)**
  BPH usually arises in central zone.
- Therefore TURP done for BPH is not protective against cancer.

Prostate cancers usually present as following types.

1) Microscopic latent type found on :
   - Autopsy
   - Specimen of Cystoprostatectomy
2) Incidently found after TURP on histopathological assessment.

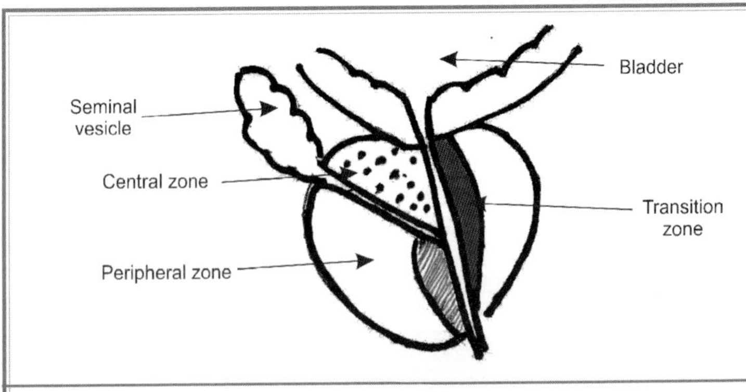

Fig. 18.1: Ca in peripheral zone

3) Found on screening by PSA.
4) Easily palpable localised Ca.
5) Locally advanced prostate Ca.
6) Metastatic disease from clinically evident prostate Ca or Occult prostate Ca.

ETIOLOGY :

- Advancing age
- High fat diet, high in red meat
- Positive family history
- Low Vit. D, High Calcium
- Obesity

PROTECTIVE :

- Selenium
- Vit. E
- Fish
- Omega-3-fatty acids

Molecular genetics :
- RNASEL
- MSR-1
- BRCA 1/2

PATHOLOGY :

a) Epithelial :

- Adenocarcinoma
- Squamous cell Ca
- Adenosquamous Ca
- Adenoid cystic Ca

- Endometroid Ca
- Comedo Ca
- Transitional Cell Ca
- Mucinous Ca
- Signet ring Ca
- Neuroendocrine Ca

b) Non-epithelial

M/C : **Adeno Carcinoma**

- Hyperchromatic enlarged nucleus with prominent nucleoli.
- Abundant cytoplasm (hence Nuclear : Cytoplasmic ratio not important).
- Basophilic cytoplasm.
- Absence of Basal cell layer - proved by IHC – HMWK normally present in basal cells will be negative in Ca.

Precursor lesions :

- PIN (Prostatic Intraepithelial Neoplasm) : increased cellular proliferation with in ducts/glands with retained basal cell layer.
- ASAP (atypical small acinar proliferation).

SCREENING for prostate Ca :

Includes : DPRE (digital per rectal examination) + Serum PSA level

- Cancer detection rate by PSA : 2-4%
- 30% with increase Prostate Specific Antigent (PSA) will have Prostate Ca on biopsy.
- 20% of patient with prostate Ca will have normal PSA.
- Many such tumours do not progress in life time.

TUMOUR SPREAD :

1. Locally :

- Upwards to involve Bladder Trigone. Further upward extension will block ureter leading to Anuria.
- Distally to involve sphincter mechanism.
- Penetration of prostate capsule is common.
- Involves seminal vesicles in advanced disease.
- Rectal involvement rare because of Denovilliers Fascia (this barrier is largely one way allowing spread of cancer from rectum to prostate but not vice versa).

2. Lymphatic :

- Obturator nodes.
- External iliac lymph nodes.

3. Hematogenous :

- Particularly to bone.
- ***Prostate** is M/C site of origin for skeletal mets followed by breast.
- M/C bone involved :
  a) Lower lumbar
  b) Pelvic
  c) Femoral head
  d) Rib cage
  e) Skull
- Mets are usually Osteoblastic/osteosclerotic.

SIGNS/SYMPTOMS :

a) Symptoms of Bladder Outflow Obstruction (BOO) implies tumour is locally advanced.

b) Pelvic pain.

c) Hematuria.

d) Renal failure resulting from obstruction.

e) Bony mets causes Bone pain, malaise, arthritis, Anaemia, Pancytopenia.

Symptoms of cord compression, pathological fracture.

Rectal examination :

In advanced state :

- On palpation one may find : Stony hard gland, nodules, induration in part/whole of the gland.
- Obliteration of median sulcus.

INVESTIGATION :

a. Blood tests :

- Pancytopenia : In metastatic condition secondary to marrow invasion.

  Anaemia may also be secondary to renal failure.
- Azotemia (tumour at trigone causing BOO +/- bilateral ureter obstruction).
- Increased Alkaline phospatase – In bone mets.
- Increased acid phosphatase suggests disease spread out of prostate
- ***Prostate specific antigen (PSA) :***
  - ➢ It is a Serine protease.
  - ➢ Conditions in which it is raised
    - ✧ BPH
    - ✧ Ca prostate
    - ✧ Urethral Instrumentation

- UTI
- Prostate infarction
- Perineal trauma
- Vigorous prostate massage

- Decrease with decrease in Serum testosterone.
- Decrease with increase in BMI
- It is mainly used to follow up course of advanced disease.
- Used for cancer screening also, however it has low sensitivity and specificity for diagnosis of localised prostate Ca
- Normal : $\leq$ 4 nmol/ml
- PSA > 10 ng/ml – Suggestive of Ca
  PSA > 35 ng/ml – Diagnostic of Ca
- Cancer detection rate by PSA : 2-4%
- 30% with - PSA will have Prostate Ca on biopsy.
- 20% of patient with prostate Ca will have normal PSA
- **Methods to improve cancer detection rate:**

1. **Estimation of molecular forms of PSA :**
   - Free
   - Bound to α1 antichymotrypsin
   - Bound to α2 macroglobulin.

   Prostate Ca demonstrate low % of free PSA compared to benign disease.
2. **PSA Kinetics :**
   - It is the rate of change of Serum PSA levels.
   - In prostate Ca this time very less.
   - Increase in serum PSA by 0.75 ng/ml/yr suggests

high risk of harboring Ca.

- PSA doubling with in < 6 months is significant.
- Significant if measured by same laboratory over period of 18 months.
- Caution: Very rapid increase is seen in prostatitis.

3. **PSA density :**
   - It is ratio of PSA level to gland volume.
   - Normal is 0.12 ng/ml/gram of prostrate tissue.

   Disadvantage :

   a) Epithelium:Stroma ratio varies from gland to gland, only epithelial component secretes PSA.

   b) Error in calculating prostate volume.

   c) Requires TRUS (invasive and uncomfortable).

- **PSA-3 :**
  - Non-coding prostate specific mRNA.
  - Over-expressed in prostatic Ca.
  - It predicts presence of Ca
  - Usefull in evaluating biopsy negative patients with rising serum PSA.

b. TRUS (Trans Rectal Ultra Sound) :

- Helps in prostatic evaluation and local Staging.
- Hypoechoic lesion in peripheral zone with hyper-vascularity/ bulging contour/angulated appearance on lateral margin suggests Ca.
- Helps in guiding biopsy/other intervention.
- Elastography – useful adjunctive to TRUS. Based on differential compressibility of Benign & malignant tissues.

c. CT/MRI of pelvis :

- Main role is for excluding LN metastasis. If enlarged LNs seen proceed with CT guided LN Biopsy.
- Not accurate for T stage.

  Accuracy can be increased by use of IV super para magnetic nanoparticles.

d. Endorectal coil MRI :

- It involves use of endorectal coil in conjunction with MR spectroscopy.
- Accuracy is better.
- Helps in locoregional characterisation & Staging.

e. Bone Scan :

- Identifies distant bony metastasis
- Not required in asymptomatic cases, T_1/T_2 cases, if PSA < 20 ng/ml

f. Antibody assisted imaging :

- Antibody against prostate specific membrane antigen conjugated to In^{111}
- Can be used for initial workup as well as staging of recurrent disease.

g. Prostate biopsy :

- ***Indication*** :
  - ➢ High Serum PSA
  - ➢ Abnormal DRE
- done under TRUS guidance.
- done under Local anasthesia (LA)/periprostatic block.
- peri-procedure antibiotic prophylaxis needed.

- It normally includes **Sextant 6 biopsies** taken along the parasagittal line to include abnormal areas on DRE/TRUS
- If Biopsy negative but suspicion is high due to raised PSA, then :

  Extended pattern biopsy – **Saturation scheme**

  To include transition zone and anterior commissure.

  20 samples taken

  2 from lateral base
  3 from lateral mid
  3 from apex
  1 from parasagittal mid
  1 from parasagittal mid

  } on either side

- **Risks** :
  - hematochezia
  - hematoma
  - hematospermia

- **Gleason Grading System :**
  - Based on appearance of glandular architecture, degree of glandular differentiation and it's relation to stroma on low power of microscope.
  - 2 grades allotted to give gleason score
    - Primary grade : Pattern of architecture that is most commonly observed.
    - Secondary grade : Pattern 2nd most commonly observed.
  - Gleason grade : 1-5

    Gleason score : 2-10

- Grade 1 & 2: Small uniform shaped glands closely packed which little intervening stroma.

  Grade 3: Variable sized gland that percolates through normal stroma in between normal glands (Cookie cutter appearance).

  Grade 4: Incomplete gland formation.

  Grade 5: Only infiltrating cells with no gland formation.

- **Score :** 2-4 – Well differentiated

  5-7 – Mod differentiated

  8-10 – Poorly differentiated

STAGING :

TNM Classification :

T1 – T1a : $\leq$ 5% of tissue in TURP specimen positive for Ca, normal DRE.

T1b : > 5% of tissue in TURP specimen positive for Ca, normal DRE.

T1c : Ca in patient with high Sr. PSA, normal TRUS, normal DRE.

T2 – T2a : Palpable on DRE, visible on TRUS involving less than ½ of one lobe.

T2b : Palpable on DRE, visible on TRUS involving more than ½ of one lobe.

T2c : Palpable on DRE, involving both lobes on TRUS.

T3 – T3a : infiltrating outside prostatic capsule

T3b : Invading seminal vesicle

T4 : Invading bladder, sphincter

N1 – : Regional LNs involved.

M1– M1a : Non regional LN involved

M1b : Bony osteoblastic metastasis

M1c : Involves other extra prostratic sites

TREATMENT :

1. **T1a** : Regular follow up with DRE and PSA for early identification of disease progression.

2. **T1b, T1c, T2** : Treatment depends upon
   a) Age
   b) Performance status
   c) Patient preference

> 70 years

Conservative TURP/stenting for Obstructing Ca with/without hormone therapy

< 70 years

if life expectancy is > 10 years

if PSA < 20 nmol/L with no metastasis

↓

Radical prostatectomy

↓

Side Effects : Incontinence : T/t artificial sphincter

Impotence: can be prevented by attempting to preserve neuro-vascular bundle

- ***Other option :***

➢ **Brachytherapy :** for low volume T1 disease.

Radioactive seeds of Iodine-125 or palladium-103 placed in prostate via transperineal needle.

- **External Beam Radio Therapy :** Radical radiotherapy, For T_1 & Low volume T_2 disease results similar to Radical prostatectomy

  Side effects : Bladder irritation, urge incontinence, Radiation proctitis

3. **T_3, T_4 :** Androgen ablation
   - Medical
   - Orchidectomy

- **LHRH agonist** : Leuprolide, Goserelin, Buserelin
- This will slow down disease progression
- 3 monthly depot injections to be given
- During initial few days it increases testosterone levels, therefore to give Antitestosterone during initial course (Bicalutamide, Flutamide, Cyproterone acetate)
- In patients aged < 70 years, one can consider Radical Radiotherapy

4. **Metastatic disease :**

- Holds Poor prognosis
- If symptomatic – Androgen Ablation
- For painful bony mets
  - Radiotherapy (if localised)
  - IV strontium - 89 (in multiple mets) (Bone seeking isotope that delivers effective radiotherapy to metastatic area)
- Systemic chemotherapy – docetaxel in young fitter patients.

✡✡✡

Chapter 19

Penile Cancer

- Constitutes < 1% of all cancer
- Seen in 6th decade of life

ETIOLOGY :

a) Poor hygiene

b) Smegma under fore skin → chronic inflammation → Cancer

c) Virus : HPV 16 (M/C)

- Circumcision decreases risk of penile Ca

PATHOLOGY :

a. **Precancerous lesion :**

1) Acanthosis
2) Leukoplakia
3) Hyperkeratosis
4) Parakeratosis
5) ***Balanitis Xerotica Obliterans :***
   - Uncommon
   - The pliant foreskin becomes thickened & whitish forming a constricting band that prevents foreskin retraction causing difficulty in maintaining hygiene
   - It may progress to cause – meatal stenosis, urethral stricture, Recurrent Balanitis,

   Treatment : Circumcision

   In early stages – topical steroids

6) ***Giant Condyloma accuminata/Buschke Lowenstein disease***

- ➢ Histology like that of verrucous carcinoma.
- ➢ It is invasive and locally destructive → water can perineum
- ➢ does not spread to lymph nodes
- ➢ does not metastasize
- ➢ caused by HPV.

Treatment : excision

7) ***Balanoposthitis :***

- ➢ Inflammation of glans & prepuce.
- ➢ **Associated with :** Lichen planus, Psoriasis, Drug hypersensitivity, Monilial infection, Diabetes, Phimosis.

b. Carcinoma in Situ :

- ***Terminology :***
  - ➢ If it involves Glans - Erythroplasia of Querat
  - ➢ If it involves Shaft - Bowen's disease

  } SCC in Situ
- Clinically it presents as a Red cutaneous patch.
- If in doubt - Biopsy: Hyperplastic cells in disordered array with vacuolated cytoplasm with mitotic figures.

c. Invasive Carcinoma :

1) **Squamous Cell Ca :** M/C type

- ➢ ***M/C Site :*** Glans → Prepuce → Shaft
- ➢ Grossly: Ulcero-proliferative
- ➢ It usually grows to gradually involve glans f/b prepuce f/b shaft

- **Buck's fascia** act as barrier to Corpora invasion & Haematogenous spread

- ***Variants/Subtypes :***

a) Verrucous Ca : Papillary appearance

b) Warty Ca (verruciform) } Associated with HPV-16 infection

c) Basaloid }

2) **Malignant melanoma :**

- Uncommon.
- Blood borne metastasis is more common.
- Treatment principle same as that for SCC.

3) Basal cell Ca

4) Paget's disease : Adenocarcinoma

5) Kaposi Sarcoma (Radiosensitive).

LYMPH NODE SPREAD : (Fig. 19.1)

Glans – Deep inguinal LN/LN of cloquet → Pelvic lymph node

Prepuce & Shaft – Superficial inguinal LN → Pelvic lymph node

Pelvic lymph node → Metastasis

If femoral node gets involved →

Femoral vessel erosion/haemorrhage

Skin necrosis

Infection

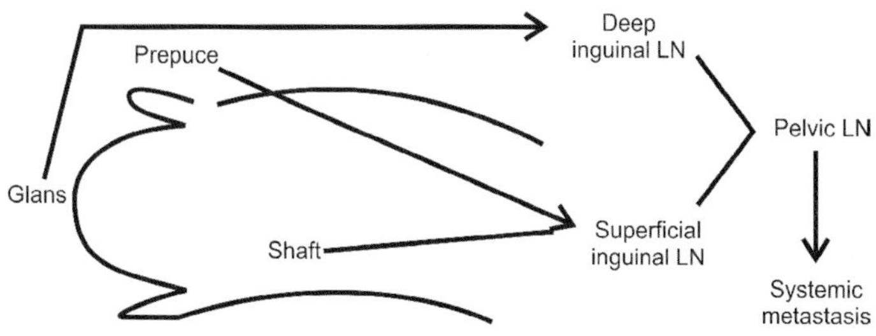

Fig. 19.1: Lymph Node Spread

SIGNS/SYMPTOMS :

a) - Non-healing ulcer – erythematous/indurated
   - Small nodule
   - Exophytic growth

b) Discharge

c) Associated with pain

d) Associated with irritative voiding symptoms

INVESTIGATIONS :

- CBC – Anaemia, leukocytosis (as penile Ca prone to infection)
- Non-metastatic hypercalcemia

IMAGING :

- X-ray chest
- CT (Abdomen + Pelvis)
- If symptomatic : Bone scan

} to rule out metastatis

D/D :

a) Syphilitic ulcer – Painless

b) Hemophilus ducryi – Painful

c) Condyloma acuminate – Exophytic, soft

BIOPSY : For establishing diagnosis.

STAGING :

AJCC's TNM staging system used :

Tis – Carcinoma in situ

T_1 – Confined to subepithelial connective tissue

T_{1a} – No lymphovascular invasion

T_{1b} – Lymphovascular invasion present

T_2 – Involvement of corpora cavernosa and spongiosa

T_3 – Involvement of Urethra

T_4 – Involvement of Adjacent structure

N_1 – Single superficial inguinal LN involved, mobile

N_2 – U/L or B/L multiple Superficial inguinal LN involved, mobile

N_3 – Fixed superficial LN or Involvement of deep/pelvic LN

M_0, M_1 – Metastasis present

TNM Staging :

Stage O – Tis, Ta

Stage I – T_{1a}

Stage II – T_{1b}, T_2, T_3

Stage III – T_1 – T_3 with N_1, N_2

Stage IV – T_4, N_3, M_1

Jackson Staging :

Stage I – Tumour confined to glans & prepuce

Stage II – Tumour involving shaft

Stage III – Tumour associated with operable inguinal LN pathy

Stage IV – extends beyond shaft,
Inoperable LN pathy
Distant mets

TREATMENT :

Stage wise treatment :

1. CIS :

a) 5-FU application
b) Imiquimod 5% - topical immune response modifier
c) Nd-yag laser therapy
d) CO_2 laser therapy
e) Cryosurgery
f) Surgical excision
g) Mohs microsurgery –
   - Layer by layer removal of tumour with immediate histopathological examination for e/o malignancy.
   - Frequent follow up necessary to monitor for recurrence.

2. Stage I :

- Tumour confined to glans, prepuce & distal shaft
- If limited to foreskin ➢ Circumcision
- If glans/distal shaft ➢ Partial penectomy with 2 cm margin
  ➢ Mohs microsurgery

   - Radiation therapy (external beam radiotherapy or Brachytherapy)

- If HPE shows high grade Ca or poor differentiation

↓

Sentinel Lymph Node Biopsy (SLNB)

↓ If -ve — Observation

↓ If +ve — B/L Ilio-inguinal LN dissection

3. **Stage II :**

   - Involving corpora/urethra without LN involvement

Partial penectomy with 2 cm margin followed by SLNB

↓ If –ve → Observation → If become palpable over a period of time → U/L Ilio-Inguinal node dissection

↓ If +ve → B/L Ilio-inguinal LN dissection

4. **Stage III :** ***(associated with operable LNpathy)***

   - 50% time palpable LN in these patients will be due to infection

Partial penectomy
↓
4-6 weeks of antibiotic therapy
↓

- LNs Disappear
  - ↓ SLNB
    - -ve → Observe
    - +ve → B/L Ilio-Inguinal Node dissection
- Persistent LNs
  - ↓ B/L Ilio Inguinal Node dissection

5. **Stage IV: (Inoperable LN, spread to entire/beyond shaft, distant mets)**
   - Palliative surgery for local penile lesion:
     Total amputation of penis with perineal urethroplasty
   - Radiation therapy for primary tumour/Lympadenopathy/bone mets
   - Chemotherapy's role is under evaluation
     - May be effective both as adjuvant or neo-adjuvant
     - Drugs : Bleomycin, methotrexate, cisplatin, 5-FU (BMC-F)

- Recurrent disease – Salvaged by penile amputation
- 5 year survival and prognosis depends on nodal disease
- Lymphadenectomy holds significant morbidity of infection, skin necrosis, wound breakdown, chronic oedema.

✡✡✡

NOTES

SECTION IV
Endocrinological Oncology

Chapter 20

Carcinoma Breast

- M/C cancer in females worldwide.
- 2nd M/C cause of cancer related death in women.
- M/C type of CA breast : Adenocarcinoma of the Invasive ductal carcinoma type.
- M/C site : Upper outer quadrant (left > right).

ETIOLOGY :

1) Hormonal factor :

   Increased estrogen exposure :

   - Early menarche, nulliparity, late 1st pregnancy, late menopause, all these increase the number of menstrual cycles & hence estrogen exposure.
   - Hormone replacement therapy (HRT)
   - Oral contraceptive pills (OCP)

2) Protective factors : increased period of lactation

   - Multiple pregnancies, Early child bearing.
   - Terminal breast differentiation occurs with full term pregnancy which is protective.

   Because of the above factors, incidence is low in developing countries.

3) Obesity
4) Diet with high fat content
5) Alcohol
6) Radiation
7) Family history
8) Genetic factors : BRCA1 & BRCA2 mutation

Cancer Genetics :

BRCA 1 & BRCA 2 mutation :

- Both are tumour suppressor genes found on chromosome 17 & 13.
- 10% of Breast Ca are due to inherited germ line mutation occurring in an autosomal dominant pattern with varying penetrance.

BRCA 1	BRCA 2
➢ Chr 17	Chr 13
➢ Increased risk bilaterally	Increased risk bilaterally
➢ Early onset	Early onset
➢ Invasive Ductal Ca	Invasive Ductal Ca
➢ Poorly differentiated	well differentiated
➢ HR (hormone receptor) Negative	usually positive
➢ Ovarian, colon, prostate Ca too	Ovarian, colon, prostate Ca & Male Breast Ca too

Hereditary risk said to be present if :

- 2 or more members of a family have developed Breast/ ovarian Ca before the age of 50 years.
- Male Breast Ca.
- Breast & ovarian Ca in same female.

Steps in genetic testing :

4 step process :

a) Detailed family history of both paternal & maternal side
b) Assess appropriateness of testing
c) Counselling consent & testing
d) Interpret Result.

- Testing done with gene sequence Analysis. First test the affected member for BRCA mutation.
- If found, all other members of the family tested for the specific identified mutation.
- In other family members :
  - If positive : Increased risk for Ca
  - If negative : Same risk as general population
- If patient has mutation but develops sporadic Ca the phenomenon is called : *Phenocopy*

Risk management :

1) Prophylactic Mastectomy with reconstruction.
2) Prophylactic oophorectomy with HRT.
3) If patient defers surgery : Intensive surveillance from Age of **25** :
   - 6 monthly Breast Examination
   - Yearly mamography
   - Yearly transvaginal US
   - Yearly Ca-125
4) Chemo prevention with Tamoxifen :
   - However Ca in BRCA 1 mutation is High grade,
   - Often HR negative,
   - Even the DCIS is HR negative

Other genetics predisposers :

- Li fraumeni Syndrome : P53
- Cowdens Syndrome : PTEN

RISK ASSESSMENT for Ca breast :

- **Gail model :**
  - Age at menarche
  - Number of Benign Breast disease/Breast biopsies
  - Age at 1st Live Birth
  - No of affected family members
- **Clauss Model :** Incorporates more information on family History.
- However neither of the two include other risk factors including BRCA 1 & 2 mutation.

- **Risk management :**
  - Decisions affected by Risk.
    - Use of HRT : because HRT increases Ca risk by 3 times
    - Age at starting screening mammography
    - Need for prophylactic mastectomy.
    - Need for tamoxifen
  - If High risk :
    - Do not use HRT
    - Tamoxifen if gail risk > 1.7
  - Side effects of tamoxifen :
    - Thrombo embolism
    - Endometrial Ca
    - Cataract
  - Alternative → Raloxifen
    - Decreased risk of Ca with reduced side effect
    - However no effect on DCIS, LCIS

Natural History :

- **Primary tumour** shows desmoplastic reaction with cancer growth
  ↓
  Skin tethering due to coopers ligament involvement
  ↓
  Disruption of dermal lymphatics
  ↓
  Peau de orange appearance
  ↓
  Ulceration
  ↓
  Satellite involvement

- **Axillary LN spread: (Most imp Prognostic Correlate)**
  - Firm hard, initially mobile, later fixed forming a Conglomerate mass.
  - Level I → III
    level I : Below or lateral to pectoralis minor : includes anterior, posterior, lateral LNs
    level II : Behind pectoralis minor : Central
    level III : Medial or above pectoralis minor : Apical

- **Distant Metastasis :** With 20th cell division (approximate tumour size : 0.5 cm) it neovascularizes
  From this moment onwards :
  - It may spread to pleura and lungs via intercostal & axillary vessels
  - To Vertebra via Batsons plexus
  - Other sites : Bones, Liver.

PATHOLOGY :

Minimal Breast Carcinoma includes : DCIS, LCIS & Invasive Ca < 0.5 cm in size.

a. **Carcinoma in situ (CIS) :**

- No invasion of basement membrane
- It may be ductal CIS or lobular CIS

LCIS	DCIS
➢ From terminal duct-lobular unit	From minor ducts
➢ Only in females	Can be seen in males
➢ Incidence: Less than DCIS	More common
➢ Sign/Symptoms :	
Usually asymptomatic	Mass, pain, discharge
➢ Calcification :	
Typically in adjacent tissue This is unique to LCIS	Micro calcification is characteristic
➢ Commonly Bilateral (B/L)	Less commonly B/L
➢ Commonly multicentric (MC)	Less commonly MC
➢ It is a Marker for increased risk	it is a Precursor lesion
➢ Risk of Subsequent Ca :	
Less compared to DCIS	more
➢ Type of Subsequent Ca	
Invasive Ductal Ca	Invasive Ductal Ca
➢ Ca tends to be bilateral irrespective of the site of LCIS	Ca lateralises to the site of DCIS

- **Microscopy :**

1. **LCIS :** Distortion & destruction of terminal duct-Lobular unit with distinctive cytoplasmic mucoid globules.

2. **DCIS :** Hyper proliferating epithelium in minor ducts

↓

Papillary pattern

↓

Cribriform pattern

↓

Solid pattern

↓

Comedo pattern (necrosis)

↓

Calcium deposition

↓

Microcalcification

- DCIS is classified based on nuclear grade & amount of necrosis into :
  High, intermediate & low risk
- **Van Nuys prognostic index** (VNPI) is widely used to classify DCIS

b. **Invasive Carcinoma :**

1) ***Paget's disease :***

- Clinically : Chronic eczematous eruption involving nipple which may progress to form a weeping ulcerative lesion
- Associated with extensive DCIS which progresses to Invasive Ca.
- Pathognomic paget cells (pale vacuolated cells) are seen in epidermal Rete Pegs.

- Differentiated from pagetoid melanoma by IHC :
  - Pagets Disease → CEA positive
  - Melanoma → S 100 positive

2) ***Invasive Ductal Ca/Non specific type (NST)/Schirrous simplex***

- 50-60 years peri/post menopausal
- M/C type, almost 80% of all breast ca
- Solitary firm mass with axillary LN metastasis being very common
- Cut section : stellate configuration with radial chalky white streaks
- HPE : glandular pattern

3) ***Medullary type :***

- Frequent phenotype of BRCAI mutation
- Frequently HR negative & B/L
- Frequently associated with DCIS
- Bulky, haemorrhagic, necrotic, soft
- HPE : Large pleomorphic cells with absence of ductal pattern with lymphocytic infiltration

4) ***Mucinous type :***

- Seen in elderly.
- Soft gelatinous tumour.
- HPE : Pool of extracellular mucin with low grade Ca cells within.

5) ***Tubular type :***

- Small

- Frequently type identified on screening mammography.
- Good survival.

6) ***Papillary type :*** usually < 3 cm
   - Less axillary LN spread
   - Good survival

7) ***Cribriform type*** → good survival

8) ***Invasive Lobular Ca :***
   - 10% of all breast ca
   - Multifocal (multiple tumour within single quadrant or within 4 cm of each other),
   - Multicentric (involving > 1 quadrant, or > 4 cm away),
   - B/L
   - HPE :
     - Histologic hallmark : tumor cells tends to invade as linear strands (Indian file pattern).
     - Cell contains mucin which displaces nucleus → Signet ring configuration.

Molecular classification :

One of the most exciting aspects of breast cancer biology has been its recent subdivision into at least five subtypes based upon gene expression profiling :

- Luminal A : ER and PR positive, Her-2 negative
- Luminal B : ER, PR and Her-2 positive: Triple positive
- Normal breast-like : Well-differentiated, ER-positive
- Basal cell type : Triple negative
- Her-2 type : Her-2 positive, ER and PR negative

SIGNS/SYMPTOMS of breast Ca :

1) Painless Lump :
   - ➢ with/without nipple discharge or nipple retraction.
2) Breast Asymmetry/Enlargement.
3) Ulceration with erythema.
4) Axillary mass.

DIAGNOSIS :

1. Local examination :

- ***Inspection*** : Size, shape symmetry, enlargement, lump, skin, nipple.
- ***Palpation*** : Size, shape, surface, location, consistency, margins, fixity, axillary LNs.

2. Mammography :

- Radiation exposure is only 0.1 cgy/study which is low, therefore no increased risk.
- It may be used for :
  - ➢ Screening : to detect unexpected Breast Ca in Asymptomatic patients.
  - ➢ Diagnostic : to evaluate women with Abnormal finding such as mass, discharge.
  - ➢ Guiding : needle localisation & biopsy.
- ***Views :***
  - ➢ Most common : Cranio-caudal (CC), Medio-lateral-oblique (MLO)
  - ➢ CC : Medial breast well visualised
  - ➢ MLO : Maximum amount of breast visualised including upper outer quadrant.

- 90 degree lateral → helps Lateralisation
- Spot compression → helps better define the lesion

- *Newer techniques :*
  - Digital mammography → allows to manipulate contrast
    - Better definition, useful in dense Breast.
  - Xeromammography → on Xerography plate
    - Positive image
    - Helps visualise both breast tissue & soft tissue of chest wall.
- *Finding in malignancy :*
  - Ill defined, irregular, stellate, spiculated margins with Microcalcification
  - High density, heterogeneous with wide halo
- **BIRADS (Breast Imaging Reporting And Data System) :**

  Category :

  0 : Incomplete assessment, need additional imaging evaluation

  1 : Negative, routine yearly mammogram recommended

  2 : Benign findings, routine yearly mammogram recommended

  3 : Probably benign findings, short term follow-up suggested

  4 : Suspicious abnormality, biopsy to be considered

  5 : Highly suggestive of malignancy, appropriate to be taken

  6 : Known biopsy-proven malignancy

3. Sono mammography :

- Helps differentiate Solid vs. Cystic lesions.

- Helps in Characterisation

  Benign→ smooth round/oval

  Malignant → irregular
- Helps Guide Biopsy
- Not good for lesions < 1 cm

4. MRI :

Usefull in : Young female with dense Breast with h/o familial Ca or genetic mutation.

5. Ductography :

- Indication : nipple discharge.
- Findings :
  - Papilloma → filling defect
  - Ca → irregular mass

6. Breast Biopsy :

- Palpable mass : → FNAC

  → Core biopsies
- Non-palpable lesion → FNAC/core biopsy under USG/Stereotactic guidance.
- Rarely open biopsy after needle localisation.
- If biopsy comes negative but high suspicion remains : Image guided biopsy/open biopsy.

Triple Assessment includes a combination of clinical assessment, radiological imaging (USG/Mammography) and tissue sampling (FNAC/Biopsy).

- The positive predictive value of Triple Assessment should exceed 99.9%.

SCREENING Guidelines :

1) $\geq$ 20 years : 3 yearly Clinical Breast Examination.
2) Baseline mammography @ 35 year.
3) Yearly mammography 40 years onwards.

STAGING : As per AJCC

- 7th AJCC TNM Staging is used for Breast Cancer.

T1 : Tumour < 2 cm

T2 : Tumour > 2 cm and < 5 cm

T3 : Tumour > 5 cm

T4a : Extension to chest wall, not including pectoralis muscle

T4b : Skin edema (including peau d'orange) or ulceration of skin, or satellite skin nodules confined to the same breast

T4c : Both T4a and T4b

T4d : Inflammatory carcinoma.

N1 : Metastasis to movable ipsilateral axillary LNs.

N2a : Metastasis in ipsilateral axillary LNs which is fixed or matted.

N2b : Metastasis in clinically apparent ipsilateral internal mammary LNs in the absence of clinically evident axillary LNs metastasis.

N3a : Metastasis in ipsilateral infraclavicular LNs.

N3b : Metastasis in ipsilateral internal mammary LNs and axillary LNs.

N3c : Metastasis in ipsilateral supraclavicular LNs.

M0 : No distant metastasis.

M1 : Distant metastasis.

Stage I : T1

Stage II : T2, T3, N1

Stage IIIA : N2

Stage IIIB : T4

Stage IIIC : N3

Stage IV : M1

- **Bloom-Richardson Grading :**

  Based on (TNM) :

  1. Tubule formation
  2. Nuclear pleomorphism
  3. Mitotic count

PROGNOSIS :

- Single most important predictor of survival is number of LNs positive.

- **Biomarkers :**

  1) Risk factor Biomarker :
     - ➢ Germline mutation, mammographic densities
     - ➢ Proliferative disease with atypia
  2) Exposure markers → DNA adducts
  3) Prognostic & predictive markers

a. Index of proliferation :

- ➢ PNCA - Proliferating cell Nuclear Antigen
- ➢ K167
- ➢ Both associated with poor grade

b. ***Apoptotic Index :***

Bax : BCL-2 ratio → Pro / Anti apoptotic

Decreased ratio → Poor prognosis

c. ***Index of Angiogenesis :***

- VEGF → Rx Bevacizumab

d. ***Index of growth factor :***

- EGFR → Her-2-neu : - Suggests poor prognosis
  - Testing to be done in all cases
  - Therapy: Transtuzumab

e. ***Steroid Hormone Receptors :*** ER (estrogen receptor)
PR (progesterone receptor

- Both positive : good prognosis
- One positive : intermediate prognosis
- Both negative : bad prognosis
- Therapy Tamoxifen
- Testing can also be assessed in FNAC & Trucut specimen
- HR testing must always be done preferentially prior to surgery

- **Nottingham Prognostic Index (NPI) :**

  Based on :

  - Tumour size in cm
  - Tumour grade
  - LN stage

  Used to select patients for adjuvant treatment.

TREATMENT :

Stage wise treatment.

1. **Early Invasive Breast Cancer (Stage I, IIA, IIB) :**

   Mastectomy + Axillary LN status assessment.

   OR

   Breast conservation therapy (BCT) + Axillary LN status assessment + RT.

   - Axillary LN status assessment may be either sentinel LN OR axillary LN dissection (Level I+II).
   - If sentinel LN cannot be identified or found to harbor metastatic disease, axillary LN dissection (Level I+II) should be done.

2. **Locally Advanced Breast Cancer (Stage IIIA, IIIB, IIIC) :**

   - Neoadjuvant chemotherapy + modified radical mastectomy (MRM) + Adjuvant RT.
   - BCT may be attempted for IIIA with N_1 with patients who achieve good response to neoadjuvant chemotherapy.
   - Systemic chemotherapy + radiotherapy are indicated in treatment of grossly involved internal mammary nodes (N3b).

3. **Distant Metastases (Stage IV) :**

   - Prolong survival and improve quality of life.
   - Hormonal therapies are preferred to cytotoxic therapy as it is associated with minimal toxicity.

- **Indications of adjuvant chemotherapy :**

1. LN positive.

2. Tumour > 1 cm
3. LN negative, > 0.5 cm with adverse prognostic factors :
   - Blood vessel or lymph vessel invasion
   - High nuclear or histologic grade
   - Her-2-neu over expression
   - Negative hormone receptor status

- ***Older regimens :***
   - CMF (Cyclophosphamide, methotraxate and 5-fluorouracil).
   - CAF (Cyclophosphamide, Adriamycin and 5-fluorouracil).

- ***Newer :***
   - AC : Adriamycin (doxorubicin) and cyclophosphamide.
   - ACT : AC plus a taxane (docetaxel, paclitaxel).

- Tamoxifen should be given for hormone receptor positive, cancer > 1 cm

  Dose : 10 mg BD X 5-years.
- Transtuzumab should be given for Her-2-neu positive cancer
- New Drugs in CA Breast :

  Ixabepilone, Lapatinib, Sunitinib.

- **Indications of Radiotherapy in Carcinoma Breast :**
   - Locally Advanced Breast Cancer (to decrease recurrence rate).
   - After breast conservation surgery.
   - Margin is positive after mastectomy.

➢ Metastases to 4 or more lymph nodes.

SURGERIES :

Types of Mastectomy :

- Simple or Total mastectomy : Removal of breast tissue, nipple-areola complex, and skin.
- Extended simple mastectomy : Simple mastectomy + removal of level I axillary LNs.
- Modified radical mastectomy : Removes all breast tissue, nipple-areola complex, skin and level I and II axillary LNs Pectoralis major is spared.

  Variants of MRM :

  a) *Auchincloss Procedure :* Removes all breast tissue, nipple-areola complex, skin and level I and II axillary LNs.

  b) *Patey's Procedure :* Pectoralis minor is removed to allow complete dissection of level III axillary LNs.

  c) *Scanlon's modification of Patey's procedure :* Pectoralis minor is divided instead of removing. Division of pectoralis minor allows complete removal of level III axillary LNs.

- Halstead's radical mastectomy : Removes all breast tissue and skin, nipple areola complex, pectoralis major and minor muscles and the level I, II and III axillary.

  Structures Preserved (ABC) : Axillary vein, cephalic vein, Long thoracic nerve of Bell.

Breast Conservative Surgery (BCT) :

- Involves resection of primary breast cancer with a margin

of normal appearing breast tissue, adjuvant radiation therapy with or without assessment of axillary LN status.

- Surgical procedures employed : wide local excision, lumpectomy, quadrantectomy.
- BCT is currently treatment for women with DCIS, Stage I and Stage II invasive breast cancer.

Suitable candidates for BCT :

- The cancer is solitary, with no clinical or mammographic evidence of cancer elsewhere in the breast.
- The tumour can be excised with tumor free surgical margins without producing a cosmetically unacceptable breast.
- There are no contraindications to radiation.
- The patients is willing and motivated for breast conservation.

Contraindications :

- Pregnancy
- Women with two or more primary tumors in separate quadrants of the breast or with diffuse malignant appearing micro calcifications.
- History of prior therapeutic irradiation.
- Persistent positive margins after reasonable surgical attempts.
- Collagen vascular disorders.
- Centrally located tumour.
- large pendulous breast.

✡✡✡

Chapter 21

Malignant Thyroid Disease

- < 1% of all malignancies.

CANCER GENETICS :

Oncogenes :

1) RET proto-oncogene

   a) Mutation – MEN_{2a}, MEN_{2b}, Familial MTC } MTC (medullary thyroid Ca)

   b) RET - PTC rearrangement
      - due to radiation exposure
      - Seen in young age, causes PTC (papillary thyroid Ca)

2) Ras – PTC, FTC (Follicular thyroid Ca)
3) BRAF – PTC, Anaplastic Ca
4) PPAR-8 – Follicular adenoma and Ca

Tumour Suppressor gene :

1) P53, 3) P15,
2) P16, 4) PTEN—Follicular adenoma & Ca

Syndromes associated with Non-medullary Thyroid Ca :

	Syndrome	Gene	Type of Ca
1)	Cowden syndrome	PTEN	Follicular adenoma and Ca, Hurthle cell tumour
2)	FAP	APC	PTC
3)	Werner Syndrome	WRN	PTC, FTC, Anaplastic
4)	Carney Complex Type 1	PPKARla	PTC
5)	McCune Albright Syndrome	GNAS1	PTC

CLASSIFICATION :

Papillary	(80%)
Follicular	(10%)
Hurthle Cell Ca	(3%)
Anaplastic	(1%)
Medullary	(5%)
Lymphoma	(< 1%)

STAGING for thyroid cancers

TNM Staging system used

T

T1 : < 2 cm

T2 : 2-4 cm, limited to thyroid

T3 : > 4 cm limited to thyroid or minimal extra-thyroidal invasion

T4a : any size, extending beyond capsule, to involve trachea, oesophagus, RLN

T4b : involving pre vertebral fascia, encasing carotid artery, mediastinal vessels

N : regional LN involvement

N1a : involvement of level VI cervical LN

N1b : involvement of other U/L, B/L cervical &/or mediastinal LN

M1 : distant metastasis present

1) ***For papillary and Follicular Ca :***

< 45 years

Stage I – any T, any N, M0

Stage II – any T, any N, M1

> 45 years

Stage I – T1

Stage II – T2

Stage III – T3 N1a

Stage IV – T4a N1b

T4b, any N, M0

any T, any N, M1

2) ***For medullary Ca :***

Stage I – T1

Stage II – T2, T3

Stage III – T3 N1a

Stage IV – T4a N1b

T4b, any N, M0

any T, any N, M1

3) ***For anaplastic Ca : Directly Stage IV***

Other prognostic indicators :

- ***AGES scoring system*** — *by Mayo Clinic*

  A : Age

  G : Histopathological grade

  E : Extrathyroidal invasion and mets

  S : Tumour size

- ***MACIS Scale*** – it's a post-op scale - *Modified from AGES*

  M : Metastases

  A : Age at presentation (<40/>40)

  C : Completeness of resection

I : Extrathyroidal invasion

S: Size

- ***AMES System :***

  A : Age < 40 M, < 50 F

  M : Metastasis

  E : Extrathyroidal invasion

  S : Size of tumour (< or > 5 cm)

- ***Degroot System :***

  Class I – Intrathyroidal

  Class II – Cervical node metastasis

  Class III – Extrathyroid invasion

  Class IV – Distant metastasis

Papillary Thyroid Cancer :

- Seen in iodine sufficient areas
- F:M = 2:1
- Age : 30-40 years
- M/C thyroid Ca in children
- M/C thyroid Ca in individuals exposed to radiation
- Patient presents with slow growing painless lump in neck.
- Majority are euthyroid
- Multifocal
- Lymph node metastasis is common.
- Patient may present with lateral aberrant thyroid. (Metastatic cervical LN).
- Adjacent structure (trachea, oesophagus, RLN) rarely involved Once involved - dysphagia, dyspnea, dysphonia.
- Distant metastasis uncommon.

- M/C site Lungs > bone > liver > brain.

PATHOLOGY :

- **Gross :**
  - White coloured, hard.
  - Remains flat on sectioning (benign lesions bulge).
  - Associated with calcification, necrosis and cystic changes.

- **Microscopy :**
  - Cuboidal cells with pale, abundant cytoplasm.
  - Papillary projections
  - **Orphan Annie nuclei :** Characteristic nucleus : Crowded nuclei with Grooving & intranuclear inclusions
  - Microscopic calcified deposits : **Psammoma bodies** (represent clumps of sloughed cells)

- **Variants :**
  - Mixed papillary follicular/Pure follicular variant/Tall cell/ Insular.
  - Columnar/Diffuse sclerosing/Clear cell/Trabecular/ Poorly differentiated.

- **Minimal/Occult micro-carcinoma** –
  - Tumours < 1 cm size.
  - No local invasion
  - No invasion of thyroid capsule
  - No angio invasion
  - No LN metastasis
  - Non palpable
  - Incidental finding on USG

- Associated with better prognosis

DIAGNOSIS :

- Local examination
- USG neck helps characterise the lesion.
- FNAC is diagnostic
- CT/MRI neck for cancer characterisation.
- CT chest if metastasis suspected.

STAGING :

- TNM Staging system used (described previously).

TREATMENT :

- Total or Near total Thyroidectomy + Routine B/L Central neck dissection.
- No role for frozen section.
- If Lateral LN involved – Modified radical neck dissection.
- Minimal/Occult micro-carcinoma- Unilateral thyroid lobectomy + Isthmusectomy.

PROGNOSIS : > 95% 10 year survival

Follicular Thyroid Cancer :

- Seen in iodine deficient areas
- F > M = 3:1
- Mean age : 50 years.
- Present with solitary painless nodule OR

  Long standing goitre showing recent onset sudden increase in size.
- Pain only if there is hemorrhage into the nodule.

- Cervical lymphadenopathy uncommon
- Distant metastasis common
- Hypothyroid/Euthyroid

- FNAC not reliable to differentiate follicular adenoma and carcinoma
  - Size > 4 cm, old age, male sex : suspect malignancy.
  - Presence of distant metastasis : malignant for sure.
  - LOH near the VHL locus of chromosome 3P, helps discriminate benign from malignant follicular lesion.
  - Micro RNA, miR-197, miR-364 } Upregulated in follicular thyroid Ca

PATHOLOGY :

- Presence of follicles without colloid.
- Architecture pattern depends on level of differentiation.
- Capsulated
- Malignancy confirmed by presence of
  - Vascular invasion
  - Capsular invasion

TREATMENT :

FNAC showing Follicular lesion

- Thyroid lobectomy – 80% times it is benign.
- If there is evidence of capsular invasion or lymphadenopathy.

  ↓

  Send specimen for frozen section → if +ve → Total thyroidectomy.

- If biopsy = follicular Ca → Total thyroidectomy.
- Total thyroidectomy directly – If old male with follicular lesion > 4 cm.
- Prophylactic neck dissection not required, unless LN involved.

Hurthle cell Cancer :

- Subtype of follicular thyroid Ca.
- Characterised by vascular/Capsular invasion.
- Not diagnosed on FNAC.
- Sheets of eosinophilic cells with mitochondria derived from oxyphilic cells of thyroid gland.
- Different from follicular as it is :
    - → Multifocal
    - → Bipolar
    - → Do not take up RAI
    - → Likely to metastasize to local nodes
    - → Prophylactic neck dissection required
    - → Propensity for distant metastasis
- High mortality
- TREATMENT :
    - ➢ Usually – Lobectomy + isthmusectomy
    - ➢ If e/o capsular/vascular invasion – Total thyroidectomy
      +
      Routine central neck node dissection
      OR
      Modified radical neck dissection if lateral group LN positive

Post-op management of differentiated thyroid Cancer

1) Radio Active Iodine therapy (RAI) :

- Post-op RAI therapy reduces recurrence.
- Metastatic differentiated thyroid Ca can be detected and treated by RAI.
- More sensitive than x-ray chest and CT for detecting metastasis.
- Less sensitive than Thyroglobulin (Tg).
- It's screening property is facilitated by removal of all normal thyroid tissue that competes with cancer cells for iodine uptake.
- Recommended for :
  - All Stage III & IV disease
  - Stage II tumour in patient < 45 years old
  - Stage I and II tumour in patients > 45 years old with
    - → Aggressive histology
    - → Multifocal disease
    - → Nodal mets
    - → Extrathyroid spread
    - → Vascular invasion
- Procedure :
  - T_4 therapy discontinued 6 weeks before testing.
  - Give T_3 during this period.
  - T_3 discontinued 2 weeks before test to allow TSH to rise
  - Low iodine diet during these 2 weeks.
  - Start with screening dose of 1-3 mCi of I^{123} and measure uptake 24 hours later.

- After total thyroidectomy uptake should be < 1%.
- "Hot" spot could represent residual normal thyroid tissue in neck thyroid bed.
- If after screening dose, uptake is significant therapeutic dose of I^{131} is given.

  30-100 mCi in low risk disease.

  100-200 mCi in high risk.

- If Tg raised but RAI neg : one dose of 100 mCi given followed by repeat imaging 1-2 weeks later
- If RAI scan +ve OR Tg level > 2 ng/ml } repeat RAI scan after 6-12 month till 1 or 2 negative scan obtained

2) External beam Radiotherapy :

To treat : - Unresectable, Locally invasive or Recurrent disease

- In bony metastasis :- to control bone pain

3) Chemotherapy :

- No routine chemotherapy advised
- Only tried in disseminated thyroid Ca
  - Doxorubicin – Used with external-beam radiotherapy
  - Paclitaxel

4) Thyroid hormone :

- Thyroxin :
  - As replacement therapy after total/near total thyroidectomy (to maintain Enthyroid state)
  - To suppress TSH : Therefore reducing stimuli for residual thyroid Ca cells

    Therefore reduces recurrence
- TSH maintained : at or below 0.1 uU/L

FOLLOW-UP :

- **Thyroglobulin :**
  - After total thyroidectomy expected levels are :
    < 2 ng/ml if on T_4
    < 5 ng/ml if hypothyroid
  - **IF** > 2 ng/ml: suspect metastatic disease or persistent normal thyroid tissue.
  - Tg measured initially at 6 months then annually if clinically disease free.

- **Imaging :**
  - RAI scan.
  - Cervical USG : at 6 & 12 months followed bt annually for upto 5 years.
  - If RAI & USG negative but Tg positive : FDG-PET scan may localise the disease.

Medullary Thyroid Cancer :

- Arise from parafollicular/C-cells derived from ultimobranchial bodies; concentrated superolaterally in thyroid lobes.
- From C-Cells, therefore produce Calcitonin.
- 75% Sporadic.
- 25% have inherited syndrome with alteration in RET proto-oncogene.

  MEN 2A
MEN 2B
Familial MTC } well defined genotype - phenotype correlation

- 50-60 years age, F:M = 1.5:1
- If associated with familial syndrome presents at younger age.
- It secretes :
  - Calcitonin
  - CEA
  - Calcitonin gene related peptide
  - Histaminadase
  - Serotonin
  - Prostaglandin E_2, F_{2a}

CLINICAL FEATURES :

- Presents with neck mass and palpable cervical lymphadenopathy.
- associated with pain/aching
- Local invasion – dysphagia, dysphonia, dyspnea
- Distant mets – liver, bone (osteoblastic)
  (lung mets very late)
- In extensive metastasis
  - Diarrhoea – due to increased intestinal motility, impaired electrolyte & water flux
  - Cushing Syndrome – due to ectopic ACTH production

PATHOLOGY :

Sporadic	**Familial**
Unilateral in 80%	B/L in 90%
	Multicentric
	associated with C-cell hyperplasia which is premalignant

- **Microscopy** – Sheets of neoplastic cells separated by collagen and amyloid
  - ➢ Amyloid – diagnostic finding
  - ➢ Immunohistochemistry positive for calcitonin.
    also for : - CEA
    - Calcitonin gene related peptide

DIAGNOSIS :

- ➢ History
- ➢ Physical examination
- ➢ Increased serum calcitonin/CEA
- ➢ FNAC of thyroid
- Family history important
- All new patient with MTC to be tested for :
  - → RET point mutation
  - → Pheochromocytoma
  - → Hyperparathyroidism
- Screening for patient with familial MTC done by :
  - ➢ Provocative test with pentagastrin
  - ➢ Calcium stimulated calcitonin levels
- Calcitonin – Sensitive tumour marker
  CEA – Better predictor of prognosis

TREATMENT :

- In familial cases :- Pheochromocytoma → operated first if present
- As MTC is multicentric, aggressive with no RAI uptake
  ↓
  Total thyroidectomy + B/L central neck dissection

- Modified radical neck dissection performed if :
    - If LNs palpable
    - If Tumour > 1 cm
- If unresectable/residual/recurrent tumour :- External beam radiotherapy.
    - There is No effective chemotherapy.
- Newer modality : Anti CEA monoclonal Antibody – Labetuzumab.
- Radiofrequency ablation – for treatment of liver mets.
- **Prophylactic Total Thyroidectomy** : advised in RET mutation carrier

  MEN 2A :- Before Age 6

  MEN 2B :- Before Age 1
    - If Serum Calcitonin/neck USG normal : – No neck dissection required.
    - If Calcitonin increased/USG s/o Thyroid Ca – Prophylactic central neck dissection.

FOLLOW-UP :

Annual measurement of :- Calcitonin & serum CEA levels +
History +
Physical examination
+/- USG, CT, MRI, FDG PET scan

PROGNOSIS :

- 10 year survival – 80%

  But if LN involved – 45%
- Best in Non-MEN/familial MTC > MEN 2A > Sporadic > MEN 2B

Anaplastic Cancer :

- M/C in females.
- 7th-8th decade.
- Usually presents as recent onset rapid increase in size in a long standing neck mass.

  Painful
- Tumour is often large and fixed to surrounding structure.
- Ulcerated/area of necrosis.
- Lymph nodes palpable.
- Evidence of metastatic spread may be present.

PATHOLOGY :

- **Gross :** Firm and whitish.
- **Microscopy :**
  - Sheet of cells with heterogeneity.
  - Cells – spindle shaped, polygonal, large, multinucleated cells.
  - Foci of differentiated tumour may be seen.

DIAGNOSIS :

- FNAC – may show giant and multinucleated cells.
- Incisional biopsy - to confirm diagnosis.

TREATMENT :

- Most aggressive tumour with average survival of 6 months.
- If resectable and patient young –Total thyroidectomy

  +

  Adjuvant chemo & Radiotherapy

- Isthmusectomy to relive tracheal obstruction with/without tracheostomy in advanced cases.

Lymphoma :

- Most are non-Hodgkin B-cell type.
- Chronic lymphocytic thyroiditis predisposes.
- May occur as part of generalised lymphomatous condition.
- Present as anaplastic Ca.
- Rapidly enlarging **painless** neck mass.
- May present with acute respiratory distress due to tracheal obstruction.
- Diagnosis : FNAC, core needle, open biopsy.

TREATMENT :

- Chemotherapy is main stay of treatment.
  CHOP+/-R.
- Combined Radio + Chemotherapy recommended.
- If do not respond to above regimen :- Thyroidectomy + nodal dissection.

Metastatic Ca :

- Rare site for metastasis.
- Usually from : Kidney, breast, lung, melanoma.
- FNAC helps in diagnosis.
- Treatment : Lobectomy.

✡✡✡

Chapter 22

Hyper Parathyroidism (HPT)

Primary Hyper Parathyroidism :

- F > M
- Results from parathyroid cell proliferation with resultant excess parathyroid hormone secretion independent of Ca++ levels.

  ↓

  Increased PTH

  ↓

  Increased GI absorption, increased Vitamin D production, decreased renal clearance.

  ↓

  Increased Ca++

ETIOLOGY :

1) **Genetics :**
   - ➢ MEN-1 Syndrome – Menin gene mutation
   - ➢ MEN-2A – RET gene mutation
   - ➢ Familial HPT
     - Isolated Syndrome
     - Associated with jaw tumour Syndrome with increased predisposition to Cancer
   - ➢ Sporadic cases show mutation in P53 & RB gene
2) Exposure to ionising radiation
3) Lithium

- HPT results from either :
  - Adenoma : single/multiple
  - Hyperplasia
  - Cancer

CLINICAL FEATURES :

- **Clinical Classic Pentad :**

Renal stones *Painful bones* *Abdominal groans*

Psychic moans *Fatigue overtones*

1) Renal stones : Calcium phosphate stones

   Chronic hypercalcemia also causes
   - Renal concentration impairment
     ↘ Polyuria, polydipsia, nocturia
   - HTN

2) Bone disease :
   a) Osteopenia M/C
   b) Osteoporosis
   c) Osteitis cystica fibrosa :
      - Increased bone turnover
      - Increased Alkaline phosphatase
      - Pathogenic x-ray findings :
        - X-ray hand: Subperiosteal resorption on radial side of index and middle finger.
        - X-ray skull: Mottled appearance with loss of definition between inner & outer table.
   d) Fracture more common

3) GI complication : PUD
Pancreatitis

4) CNS - PSY → Psychosis, obtundation, coma.
5) Fatigue with weakness in proximal muscle group.
6) Chondrocalcinosis, pseudogout
7) Increased risk of death from CVS disorders.

- ***Physical examination :***
  - Parathyroid lesion rarely clinically palpable unless malignant.
  - Eyes : Band keratopathy → Calcium deposition in Bowans membrane.
  - Fibro-osseous jaw tumour indicate possibility of Cancer.

D/D for Hyper Calcemia :

1) ***Malignancy :***
- Haematological – Maligant myeloma.
- Solid organ: Breast, Lung, kidney → Bone metastasis → PTH-r-P.

2) ***Endocrine :*** Hyperthyroidism

3) ***Granulomatous disease:*** Sarcoidosis, TB

4) ***Drugs :***
- Milk Alkali Syndrome
- Thiazide : Can be used for unmarking subclinical HPT
- Lithium
- Vit D & A

5) ***Immobilisation***

6) ***Familial hypocalciuric hypercalcemia :*** related to CASR gene mutation.

DIAGNOSIS :

a. Serum :

- Increased Ca
- Decreased phosphate
- Increased PTH
- Increased Alkaline phosphatase
- Hyperchloremic metabolic acidosis
- Increased 1, 25 dihydroxy Vit D

b. Urine : Normal or Increased Ca

c. Radiology :

- X-ray skull & hand
- Bone mineral density → DEXA
- Abdominal USG → kidney stone
- OGD scopy : PUD

Pre-op Localisation studies :

a. Non-invasive :

1) ^{99m}Tc Setsambi Scan → widely used. / allows SPECT.
   - *Disadvantage :* false negative common with multiple Abnormal PT
   - Should be complemented with USG
2) USG → Identifies juxta/Intra thyroidal tumour.
3) CT & MRI for identifying Ectopic PT especially in mediastinum.

b. Invasive :

1) Pre-op

- FNAC
- Angiography
- Venous sampling

2) **Intra-op :**
   - Intra-op PTH Assay - when PTH falls by 50% or greater 10 min after removal of PT tumor — positive test —— surgery terminated.
   - Intra-op ultrasound.

TREATMENT :

- Patient who have classical symptoms → Surgery.
- When Asymptomatic → conservative approach may be applied : biannual Serum Ca++, Annual BMD, Serum creatinine.
  - ➢ However consider surgery if :
    1) Calcium level > 1 mg/dl above normal.
    2) Elevated 24 hr urinary calcium excretion.
    3) Kidney stone on investigation.
    4) Previous life threatening episode of hypercalcemia.
    5) Reduced creatinine clearance.
    6) Substantially reduced BMD.
    7) Age < 50.
  - ➢ Surgery improves symptoms.
- **Conduct of surgery** (B/L neck exploration) :
  - ➢ Supine with neck extended
  - ➢ 3-4 cm incision just caudal to cricoid cartilage
  - ➢ Strap muscle divided
  - ➢ Middle thyroid vein ligated
  - ➢ Thyroid lobe retracted medially
  - ➢ Dissect between thyroid & carotid to find PT

- Normal location is : Within 1 cm of junction of RLN & Inferior thyroid artery **(Fig. 22.1).**
  - It appears as fat globule
  - If suspected globule is incised : PT gland "POP's out".
  - Alternatively used "FLOAT sign"
- To confirm a suspicious nodule : it may be aspirated with fine needle & syringe containing 1 cc of saline → to check for high PTH levels.

- **If Lower PT not found check :**
  - Thymus
  - Carotid sheath from bifurcation to base of neck
  - Intra op USG → for intra thyroidal PT

    OR Thyroid incised Post laterally

    OR Lobectomy & bread loafing done
  - ***Rarely :*** Maldescended PT may be found high up in neck or in Anterior mediastinum.

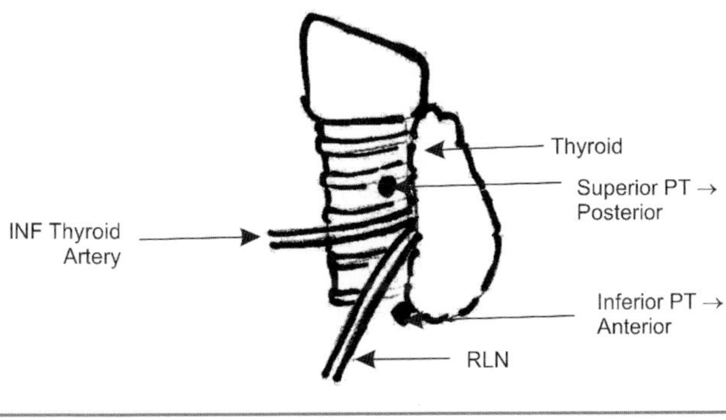

Fig. 22.1: RLN & Inferior thyroid artery

- **Upper PT has a more stable location :**

  If not found, check :
  - Carotid sheath
  - Retro esophagus
  - Tracheo esophageal groove
  - Posterior mediastinum

- ***All Attempts are made to identify all 4 glands***
  - All abnormal glands to be removed
    - Normal appearing glands can be confirmed by histology : Frozen section/Biopsy.
  - If all 4 are enlarged, hypercellular → PT Hyperplasia.

    Treatment Options :

    1) 3½ parathyroidectomy.

    2) Total parathyroidectomy & auto transplantation.

Other Approaches :

- **U/L neck exploration/focussed Approach:**
  - If both nuclear scan and USG independently identify same gland & no other → **Focussed surgery**
  - Decreased operative time & complications.
  - but risk of missing adenoma/hyperplasia in other glands as no attempt in made to locate other glands.

- **B/L neck exploration becomes a must if :**
  - If localisation studies/IO-PTH assay not available.
  - Studies fall to localise.
  - H/o syndromic disease MEN1, MEW2A, & Familial PHT.

  - Finding minimally abnormal gland on focussed surgery.

- Radio guided surgery using Tc99 setsambi
  - Useful for Redo surgery
  - Can be done under local anesthesia & sedation
  - Low Accuracy in multiglandular disease

- Endoscopic approach

✡✡✡

Chapter 23

Adrenal Disorders

Hyper Aldosteronism :

It may be :

Primary Hyper Aldosteronism/Conn's Syndrome

- Due to Autonomous secretion of Aldosterone with suppression of RAS (Renin-angiotensin system).

Secondary Hyper Aldosteronism :

- Due to RAS activation: Low flow states like, cirrhosis/CCF.

Conn's Syndrome :

- 30-50 years
- M > F
- mostly due to :
  - Adrenal Adenoma
  - B/L Idiopathic Adrenal Hyperplasia
  - Rarely Carcinoma
  - Gluocorticoid suppressible hyper aldosteronism

SIGNS/SYMPTOMS :

- Hypertension : moderate to severe.

  Long standing difficult to treat

Associated with

- Hypokalemia
- Weakness & fatigue
- Polydipsia, polyuria, nocturia

INVESTIGATION :

- Hypokalemia : < 3.2 mEq/L
  40% may be normokalemic
- Elevated plasma Aldostrone levels with suppressed plasma RAS
- Aldosterone to Renin ratio (ARR) of > 25 is suggestive of diagnosis

Sodium loading test :

- 2-3L of NS given after 5 days of low Na+ diet – measure plasma aldosterone
- Failure of fall in aldosterone level : suggestive of &
- If > 5 ng/ml : diagnostic of Conns Syndrome

LOCALISATION :

- CT } can detect Adenoma
- MRI }
- Scintigraphy with NP59 → hot nodule → Adenoma
  OR
  B/L Increased uptake → hyperplasia
- Selective venous catherisation & adrenal vein sampling after ACTH administration helps identify unilaterality
  - However it is invasive and used only in highly ambiguous cases.

TREATMENT :

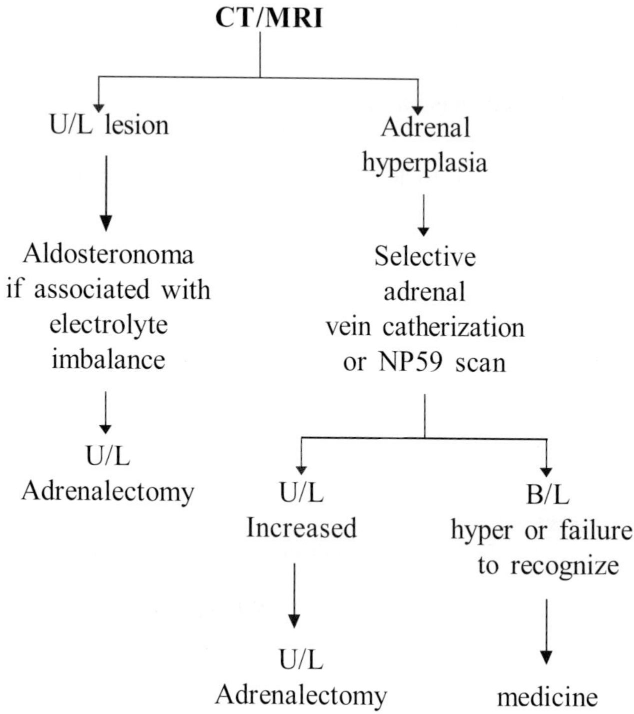

Surgery : Adenoma → Adrenalectomy < Laproscopy OR Posterior open Approach

- If Carcinoma is suspected Anterior. Trans Abdominal approach
- B/L hyperplasia : Surgery has less role
  - Benefit of surgery can be predicted by: Selective venous sampling.

Medical management : It includes :

- Aldosterone antogonist → Spironolactone
- Anti-hypertensives:
  - K+ sparing diuretic : Amiloride
    Triamterene
  - CCB : Nifidipine
  - *ACE* inhibitor : Captopril
- Gluco corticoid suppressible Hyperadenaloma: Dexamethasone

Cushing Syndrome :

Refers to symptom complex resulting from hyper secretion of cortisol regardless of aetiology.

I. ACTH Dependant :

1) Cushing Disease

- ACTH secreting pitutary
- M/C Endogenous cause adenoma

2) Ectopic ACTH production

- Carcinoid (> males)
- Bronchial adenoma (> females)

3) Ectopic CRH Production

- → Bronchial Carcinoid
- → Pheochromocytoma

II. ACTH - Independent :

- Adrenal Adenoma
- Adrenal Carcinoma

- Adrenal hyperplasia

III. Iatrogenic :

Exogenous steroid administration. M/C cause overall.

IV. Pseudo Cushing Syndrome :

Stress, major depression, alcoholism, pregnancy, chronic disease.

- **Adrenal Hyperplasia :**
  - Primary → micro/macro nodular.
  - Associated with excess ACTH → usually macronodular.
  - Primary pigmented macronodular hyperplasia may be associated with Carneys complex :

    Atrial Myxoma + schwanomma + Naevi

CLINICAL FEATURES : (Fig. 23.1)

From top to bottom :

1. Emotional liability, depression, psychosis
2. Head ache, visual disturbance
3. Moon facies
4. Hisutism
5. Hyper pigmentation
6. Buffalo Hump
7. Thin weak extremities
8. Central obesity with weight gain
9. Purple striae with plethora due to thinning of dermis
10. Amenorrhea
11. Impotence with decreased libido

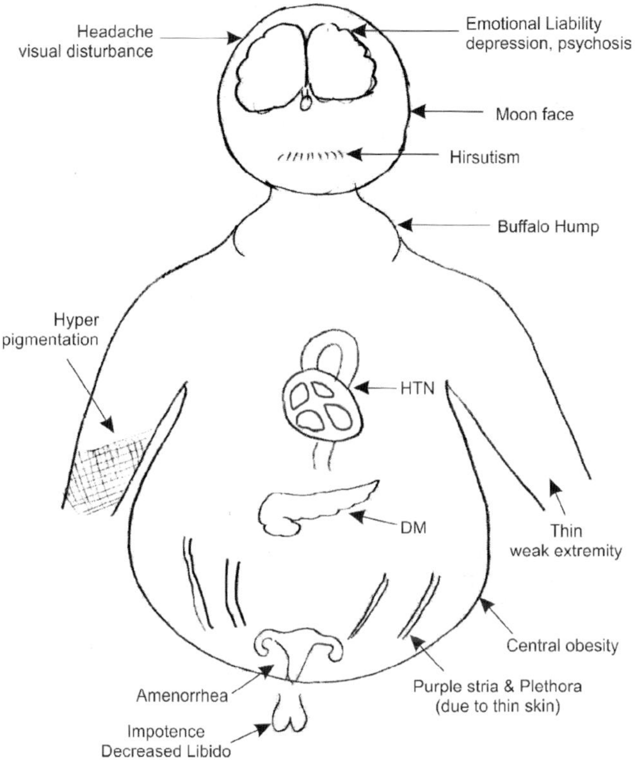

Fig. 23.1: Clinical features of cushing Syndrome

12. Hypertension, Diabetes & hyperlipidemia
13. Hypokalemia, osteopenia, polyuria

DIAGNOSIS :

a. Confirmatory tests :

- **Overnight dexamethasone suppression test** (DST) (Low dose/classic) cortisol level of < 3 mg/dL s/o other diagnosis.

- 24 hours Urinary cortisol > 100 mg/dl s/o diagnosis.
- Salivary cortisol at 11.00 pm.

b. **To determine source** (whether adrenal or extra adrenal)
- Plasma ACTH
- High dose DST
- CRH test

Scenarios :

a. Plasma ACTH :

- Increased ACTH → Cushing Disease / Ectopic ACTH production (Highest levels) / CRH producing tumour
- Suppressed ACTH → Primary Adrenal source

b. High dose DST (Pituitary vs Ectopic) :

- Suppression present → Pituitary source
- Failure to suppress → Ectopic source

c. CRH Test :

Test helps find out if a pituitary tumour may be causing Cushing's syndrome. ACTH level response to CRH administration noted

- Blunt Response → Primary Adrenal disease.
- Elevation of ACTH → pitutary disease
- Equivocal cases → Petrosal venous sampling recommended

Tests for Localisation :

- *Adrenal cause :*
  - CT/MRI : differentiate Adenoma from Carcinoma.

- MRI provides better visualisation of vascular anatomy.
- NP59 scanning

- ***Pituitary cause :***
  - CT brain.
  - Petrosal venous sampling with CRH stimulation.

- **Ectopic ACTH :**

  CT chest, check anterior mediastinum

  ↓

  If negative : CT neck

  CT Abdo + pelvis

TREATMENT :

- Adrenal tumor – ADRENALECTOMY
  - < 6 cm in size : Laparoscopic approach
  - > 6 cm in size
  - Suspicion of cancer :
    B/L Adrenal Hyperplasia

    } open Adrenalectomy

- **Pituitary tumour :**
  - Transphenoidal resection/Stereotactic radio-surgery.
  - If Ectopic source identified : treat surgically.
  - If not → palliative B/L Adrenalectomy.

- **Pre-op measures :**
  - Prophylactic Antibiotics & Anti coagulant as prone to Infection & hypercoaguation and DVT.

- **Post-op measures :**
  - In U/L tumour : IV Hydrocortisone 100 mg od x 2 years.

- As the contralateral adrenal would be suppressed.
- Therefore if replacement is not given → post op Addison's
- If B/L resection done → Lifelong Steroids + Mineralo-corticoids
- Hydrocortisone: 20 mg, 9 am – 10 mg, 9 pm
- Fludrocortisone: 0.05 mg/day

- **Unfit frail patient :**

  Medical Adrenalectomy :
  - Metyrapone
  - Aminogluthemide
  - Ketoconazole

Adrenocortical Carcinoma :

- Majority sporadic
- Syndromes Associated with it :
  - MEN 1
  - Li Fraumeni's Syndrome
  - Carneys complex
  - Beckwidt weidmann Syndrome
- 50% non-functioning

CINICAL FEATURES :

- Non-functioning : Mass, abdomen/back pain.
- Functioning → Cushing Syndrome with virilisation.

DIAGNOSIS :

a. Blood tests :

- Serum Potassium
- Urinary catecholamine levels
- DST & urinary cortisol
- 17 keto-steroid levels

b. CT, MRI :

- Size is single most important predictor of malignancy.
  > 6 cm : highly suggestive
- Other : ➢ Heterogenous
  - ➢ Necrosis & haemorrhage
  - ➢ LNs
  - ➢ Metastasis → especially to liver
  - ➢ Invasion into surrounding structures

PATHOLOGY :

Difficult to distinguish benign from malignant

- Capsular invasion most reliable sign of Carcinoma
- Other feature : ➢ Nuclear grade
  - ➢ Mitotic index

STAGING : is as per **AJCC's TNM system**

T1 : </= 5 cm in size, no extra adrenal invasion

T2 : > 5 cm in size, no extra adrenal invasion

T3 : Tumour of any size with local invasion, but not invading adjacent structures

T4 : Invading adjacent structures

N1 : LN metastasis

M1: Distant metastasis

TREATMENT :

- **Surgery :**
  - Open Adrenalectomy with En-bloc resection of contiguously involved structures
  - R_0 : good survival
  - =/>R_1 : poor survival
- Adjuvant therapy : Mitotame (Adrenolytic action)

  Also useful in unresectable stage IV tumours
- Others : Suramin, Gossypol
- **Unfit frail patient :**

  Medical Adrenalectomy
  - Metyrapone
  - Aminogluthemide
  - Ketoconazole

Pheochromocytoma :

- 50 Years
- M > F or M = F
- **10% tumour** : 10% B/L

  10% Inherited

  10% malignant

  10% in children

10% extra adrenal → from sympathetic ganglia
→ paraganglionoma
- → Organ of Zukerkandl (M/C)
- → Neck
- → Mediastinum
- → Abdomen
- → Pelvis

- It may be **Sporadic**

  OR
- **Inherited** :
  1) MEN-2, tend to be benign
  2) VHL
  3) NF 1
  4) Carney's Syndrome - GIST + paraganglionoma + Pulmonary chondroma
  5) Paraganglioma - Pheochromocytoma Syndrome, tends to be malignant

PATHOLOGY :

- Differentiating benign vs malignant is very difficult
- Even capsular invasion/nuclear grade/mitotic index not reliable
- Most reliable is
  - Invasion of surrounding structures
  - Metastasis

CLINICAL FEATURES :

Classical triad : hypertension + diaphoresis + palpitation

- Paroxysmal Hypertension: - M/C presentation.

- CVS & CNS complication - CAD, Stroke precipitating by a range of stimuli including excercise, micturition & even defecation.
- Sudden death.
- Anxiety, paresthesia, flushing.
- Chest pain, Dyspnoea.
- Abdominal pain, nausea, vomiting.

DIAGNOSIS :

- **Urine tests :**
  - ➢ Urinary Metanephrine is the most sensitive test.

  Others :
  - ➢ Urinary VMA
  - ➢ Urinary Norephinephrine, Ephinephrine, Dopamine.

- **Blood tests :**
  - ➢ Plasma Metanephrine, Norephinephrine, Ephinephrine, Dopamine and Chromogranin A
  - ➢ **Most reliable → plasma Metanephrine**
  - ➢ Adrenal vs Extra Adrenal (as only Adrenal gland has N. methyl transferase)

    ↓ ↓

    Epinephrine Norepinephrine
  - ➢ Clonidine suppression test → cannot suppress catecholamine levels in pheochromocytoma

- **Local information :**
  - ➢ CT without contrast.
  - ➢ MRI 100% sensitive (extremely bright) investigation of choice in pregnant.

- MIBG scan.

TREATMENT of choice : Open Adrenalectomy

But one has to take care to avoid rupture.

- **Pre-op measures :**

  Medical management → control BP & replete volume

  1) α Blocker : Phenoxy benzamine, given for 1-3 weeks before surgery

     - With Rehydration

     - Other α Blocker : prazosin

  2) β-blocker → propanolol after α-blockage

  3) ACE-Inhibitors & CCB

- **Intra-op :**

  BP controlled with NTG, Nitropruside & Phentolamine

  - Induction with inhalational agents: Isoflurane or Enflurane
  - Avoid stress
  - Arrythmia → Esmolol

- **Post-op :**

  Volume resuscitation to prevent hypotension resulting from loss of vasoconstrictor effect.

- **Hereditary Pheochromocytoma :**

  - U/L tumour with no evidence of tumour in opposite side : U/L Adrenalectomy
  - B/L tumour :

1) Cortical sparing Adrenalectomy : High risk of recurrence.
2) Total B/L Adrenalectomy & Autotransplantation.

Incidentaloma :

DEFINITION :

- Adrenal lesions discovered during imaging preformed for unrelated reasons excluding evaluation done for symptoms resulting from adrenal hormone hypersecretion.
- By definition it does not include : Overt Cushing Syndrome.
- But may include subclinical Syndrome with subtle clinical feature like:
  - ➢ Weight gain, facial fullness, DM, HTN
  - ➢ With loss of diurnal variation in cortisol level
  - ➢ DST positive
- It is important to identify these subclinical features because such patients may develop Addison's post-op.

Other possible diagnosis :

- Functioning : ➢ Hyper Aldosteronoma
  - ➢ Sex steroid Adrenoma
  - ➢ Pheochromocytoma
- Malignant : ➢ Pheochromocytoma
  - ➢ Adrenocortical Carcinoma
- Non-functioning : ➢ Metastasis from → Lung, Breast, melanoma
  - ➢ AC Ca

- Benign:
  - ➢ Myelo-lipoma
  - ➢ Cyst
  - ➢ Haemorrhage
  - ➢ Adenoma

INVESTIGATION :

➢ To r/o Cancer } Both require
To r/o functioning tumor } Adrenalectomy

	Benign	vs	Malignant
➢	Well encapsulated regular, Margin, homogeneous, hypo attenuating		> 6 cm, irregular margin, heterogeneous, hyper attenuating

➢ **Specific tests :**

- ***Cushing Syndrome :***
  - Low dose DST
  - 24 hour Urinary cortisol f/b
  - High dose DST & ACTH levels
  - If required CRH test

- ***Sex steroid tumours :***
  - C-17 Ketosteroid levels

- ***Pheochromocytoma :***
  - 24 hour urinary - Catecholamines, VMA, Metanephrine.
  - Plasma - Catecholamines, Metanephrine, Chromogranin A.

- *Aldosterone excess :*
    - Serum K+, Na+
    - Plasma Aldosterone & Plasma RAS activity

➢ **Local Information :**

- CT, MRI
- NP 59 scan
- MIBG scan

TREATMENT :

For functioning OR malignant tumours } Adrenalectomy

Non-functioning :

- Balance risk of surgery with risk of disease
    - ➢ > 6 cm in size : operate
    - ➢ < 4 cm : surveillance
    - ➢ 4-6 cm : controversial
    - ➢ > 4 cm < 6 cm, young fit patient → operate
- Myelolipoma per se does not warrant surgery.

  But if > 4 cm : likely to bleed surgery : operate
- Metastasis : operate

Addison's Syndrome :

Primary	Secondary
• Autoimmune • Infection : CMV, TB, • Haemorrhage following meningococcal infection : Waterhouse freiderichson Syndrome • Infiltrative disease - Amyloidosis, haemochromatosis • Metastasis • Drugs → mitotane, Aminogluthamide, ketoconazole, metyrapone • B/L adrenalectomy • Stress, trauma • Coagulopathy	• Sheehan's syndrome • Pituitary resection • Pituitary tumors

CINICAL FEATURES :

- Hypotension, fatigue, weakness, confusion.
- Abdominal pain, nausea, vomiting.
- Salt craving.
- Symptom complex mimicking: Sepsis, MI, Pulmonary Emboli.

INVESTIGATIONS :

- Decrease Na, Increase K+
- Decrease Blood sugar level
- Decreased cortisol (ACTH stimulation test)

- ACTH : Increase in primary
  Decrease in secondary

TREATMENT :

- Volume resuscitation NS & DNS.
- Cortiostroid administration:
  - Dexamethasone 4 mg
  - Hydrocortisone 100 mg
- Treat primary condition
- Mineralocorticoid may be needed

✡✡✡

Chapter 24

Carcinoma Lung

- One of the M/C cancers.
- M/C cause of Ca death.
- Limited surgical role as most present with Advanced disease.

ETIOLOGY :

1) Smoking : related to number of smoking pack years
2) Environmental pollution
3) Occupational exposure - Cadmium
4) Exposure to Radon

PATHOLOGY :

4 types :

1) Adenocarcinoma (ACA) :

- ➢ Peripherally located
- ➢ Metastasize earlier

Broncho Alveolar Ca :

- ➢ Subtype of ACA, more indolent
- ➢ Well differentiated
- ➢ Spread along alveolar wall
- ➢ Ground glass appearance on x-ray

2) Squamous Cell Ca (SCCA) :

- ➢ Centrally located
- ➢ Metastasize later
- ➢ Central necrosis & cavitation

HPR : Keratinisation & stratification
Intercellular bridge formation present

3) **Large cell Ca :**
   - ➢ Peripherally located
   - ➢ Metastasize earlier
   - ➢ Undifferentiated carcinoma
   - ➢ HPR : Anaplastic pleomorphic cells
     Neuro-endocrine histological features

4) **Small cell/Oat cell Ca :**
   - ➢ Centrally located
   - ➢ Metastasize later
   - ➢ Arise from neural crest cells
   - ➢ Very aggressive

SIGNS/SYMPTOMS :

- Cough with dyspnoea and chest pain.
  Severe localised pain suggest infiltration of intercostal nerves.
- Haemoptysis
- Weight loss
- Pleural effusion
- Clubbing
- Ca in apical Area may involve brachial plexus to cause : Pancoast Syndrome
- Advanced Ca : Dysphagia → esophagus
  Hoarseness → RLN
  SVC Syndrome → SVC

- Small Cell Ca : **Eaton Lamburt Syndrome** which is similar to Myasthenia gravis

INVESTIGATION :

- **X-ray chest :** May detect tumour.
- **HRCT :**
  - 1st investigation in suspected cases.
  - Provides locoregional stage
  - To rule out distant mets
- **PET-CT:** To rule out distant mets
- **Sputum Cytology :** High false negative rate
- **Invasive tests :**

1) Bronchoscopy : useful for evaluating centrally located tumors, allows cytological assessment.
2) Endobronchial US & EUS → Assessment & transbronchial needle aspiration (TBNA) of suspicious LNs.
3) CT guided biopsy → for peripheral tumor.
4) Mediastinoscopy, Mediastinotomy, VATS }
   - T & N stage assessment
   - Avoids unnecessary thoracotomy in advanced cases
   - Allows tissue biopsy of both primary tumour & LN

STAGING :

TNM Staging system used :

T

T1 : < 3 cm in size, within lung.

T2 : > 3 cm < 7 cm in size, invading visceral pleura.

> 2 cm away from carina.

T3 : > 7 cm in size, invading chest wall, invading mediastinal pleura, pericardium.

< 2 cm from carina.

Atelectasis of entire lung.

T4 : Involvement of mediastinal structures.

N

N1 : Ipsilateral hilar LN

N2 : Ipsilateral mediastinal, subcarinal LN.

N3 : Contralateral mediastinal, hilar LN.

Ipsi/contralateral supraclavicular, scalene LN.

M

M1
- Separate tumor in contralateral lobe.
- Pleural nodule with malignant pleural effusion.
- Distant metastasis.

WORK-UP :

Patient factors : General fitness & Lung function tests.

Spirometry & DLCO test (Diffusion capacity of Lung for Carbon monOxoide)

↓

f/b Quantitative perfusion lung scan & ^{99m}Tc labelled Albumin scan } help to assess function of residual lung that would remain after resection

↓

followed by Cardiopulmonary exercise testing.

TREATMENT :

- **Small cell/Oat cell Ca Rx :** Chemoradiation with prophylactic cranial irradiation.
- **All other types are amenable to Surgery**
- **Tumor upto : T3 N1 M1 is resectable**

Principle : R0 resection with conservation of as much lung as possible

NICE recommendations for surgery :

1) Non small cell Ca + fit for surgery → open/thoracoscopic Lobectomy
   - Surgery of choice
   - Segmentectomy/Wedge resection : for smaller tumors
2) Bilobectomy or Pneumonectomy +/- Bronchial/ vascular resection with reconstruction } When required to achieved clear margins for larger tumours
3) T3 tumours→ Neo-adjuvant chemotherapy (NACT) followed by Surgery

   Tumour with chest wall involvement: NACT followed by enbloc resection of chest wall
4) LN involvement → Enblock resection OR hilar & mediastrinal LN sampling

- **Complication of Lung resection :**
  1) Bleeding
  2) Infection
  3) Air Leak

4) Bronchopleural fistula : due to bronchial stump dehiscence

- Post-op → Physiotherapy is a must
  - Pain relief :
    - ➢ PCA : patient controlled analgesia
    - ➢ Epidural
    - ➢ Oral Analgesia
- Other Local therapy → Stereotactic Radio Surgery
- Adjuvant chemo - Radiotherapy - Improves survival
  - Platinum doublet ⟹ Carboplatin + Paclitaxel + Radiation ± Bevacizumab

✡✡✡